THE
Autism
Revolution

THE
Autism
Revolution

WHOLE-BODY STRATEGIES

FOR MAKING LIFE ALL IT CAN BE

Martha Herbert, MD, PhD

with Karen Weintraub

HARVARD HEALTH PUBLICATIONS

HARVARD MEDICAL SCHOOL

BALLANTINE BOOKS · NEW YORK

No book can replace the diagnostic expertise and medical advice of a trusted physician. Please be certain to consult with your doctor before making any decisions that affect your health or the health of your children, particularly if you or they suffer from any medical condition or have any symptom that may require treatment.

Published in the United States by Ballantine Books, an imprint of The Random House Publishing Group, a division of Random House, Inc., New York.

BALLANTINE and colophon are registered trademarks of Random House, Inc.

Library of Congress Cataloging-in-Publication Data

Herbert, Martha R.
The autism revolution : whole-body strategies for making life all it
can be / by Marth R. Herbert, with Karen Weintraub.
p.   cm.
Includes bibliographical references and index.
ISBN 978-0-345-52719-6
eBook ISBN 978-0-345-52721-9
1. Autism in children—Nutritional aspects.   2. Autism in
children—Treatment.   3. Autism in children—Psychological aspects.
4. Self-care, Health.   I. Weintraub, Karen.   II. Title.
RJ506.A9H45 2012
616.85'88206—dc23   2011044922

Printed in the United States of America on acid-free paper

www.ballantinebooks.com

246897531

First Edition

Book design by Caroline Cunningham

In memory of my parents and of Ted Carr; they would have enjoyed each other. . . .

—MRH

To the greatest children and most supportive husband anyone could ever want.

—KW

To our friends and the families whose stories we tell here, who have fought what is challenging about autism and cherished what is extraordinary about themselves and their children.

—MRH and KW

CONTENTS

PART III

Transcend Autism: Share the Strengths and Lose the Pain

From Seeing What You Believe to Believing What You See

This book is based on real stories of children and adults with autism who didn't follow the textbooks. They got better—some dramatically so. Although I changed their names and was vague on details to protect their privacy, I was meticulous in sticking to the facts of their stories and letting their experiences direct how I explained the science.

Textbooks do not include the possibility that people with autism get this much better. Neither does a lot of scientific research.

In that sense, you may say that I have gotten ahead of the science. Not everyone will be able to get such fabulous results for themselves or their child. But I have confidence that science and medicine will make these advances possible to many more people going forward.

As I have dug into current research to write this book, I have been stunned by how much science there is to support the approaches parents are taking to get their kids better. Karen Weintraub, an experienced science journalist who has shared this journey with me, has been equally amazed. Every day our Internet alerts and Listservs overflow with research publications and news stories about every area we discuss, and their findings are largely resonant with what we are explaining in this book.

There are days when we feel that there is not simply an Autism Revolution, but a global groundswell, even a tidal wave of new thinking.

FINDING COMMON GROUND

The autism world is filled with different groups that often disagree with one another. But they all make important points.

There's the neurodiversity movement, which views autism as a way of being different. People with autism have a powerful and valid way of looking at the world; it's just not the typical way.

Mainstream medicine wants treatment to be based on evidence and insists on proceeding cautiously and safely.

Advocates from the biomedical treatment world approach each person as an individual who deserves the best possible shot at maximal improvement.

There are the parents who want help for their kids—not to fight insurance companies, school districts, and doctors who don't know what they don't know.

And there are the families that have managed to leave autism behind or transcend its limitations, who offer all of us endless hope and inspiration.

This book is based on the premise that all these groups are right about their part of the picture. But the whole picture is bigger than any one part.

We can all agree that many, many people with autism are extraordinarily gifted and have much to offer the rest of us. We would all like to know precisely what is going on in the biology of autism, and provide safe and effective treatments for it. We all want new ways to relieve autism's sometimes debilitating symptoms, and to help these children learn and flourish as much as possible. We would all like to spare parents the agony of being told that there's something "wrong" with their child, of having to clean up a dozen diarrhea-filled diapers a day, and of worrying that the love of their life will never be able to say "I love you" back.

I am not just paying lip service to this idea that every major point of view has something to contribute. I genuinely believe it. And I wish more people did, too. Addressing autism is such a daunting task that all of us who care about it need to be working together, instead of arguing among ourselves. I wrote this book in the hopes of providing a framework that can integrate everyone's perspectives.

HOW TO READ THIS BOOK

Most of what I offer here are strategies I think everyone can get behind. They're safe, relatively simple, and often effective. Systems science supports my belief that small adjustments can sometimes trigger big changes. My goal is to offer parents, caregivers, and adults facing autism themselves some new ways of thinking about what they do every day and how the parts interact.

Autism is so diverse that what works for one person won't work for another; you'll have to cobble together your own distinct set of approaches. And autism is complicated, too, so no one approach is going to "fix" it. At the least, the organizing framework I suggest will help you make your child healthier and therefore better able to handle the autism symptoms that remain. The whole-body approach I'll show you dovetails with the scientifically proven behavioral therapies that are a critical part of any autism program.

Throughout the book, I address readers as if they are parents of children on the autism spectrum, but I hope that others will see themselves in the book, whether they are people on the spectrum, grandparents, pediatricians, teachers, therapists, doctors, or scientists.

This book is written in ten chapters, each framed around a different strategy or piece of the puzzle. Each chapter will include concrete advice on what you can do to help your child and/or yourself. And each chapter will tell a story meant to inspire you and show you that there are different ways to approach autism and your own reactions to it. The people I feature represent a range of ways of being autistic and a range of economic and cultural backgrounds. Many of them functioned low enough on the spectrum that no one would have predicted how well they are doing today. I am reporting here what each of these people or families thinks or did—not saying what I think they should have done. I'm not going to tell you what medications you should or shouldn't be on, and I'm not going to tell you what your doctor should do for you. That's between you and your doctor—and please do consult your doctor. Instead I'm going to provide a framework for keeping track of the whole autistic person, while you analyze the pros and cons of each new treatment or therapy that comes your way. My goal is to get you to reframe what you think you know about autism, to connect you to a larger world of autism, to turn your answers and constraints into questions, and to open possibilities.

WHAT'S NEW?

Why are my ideas about autism so different from many other people's? I think there are three answers. One, as I'll describe in the first chapter, patients in my pediatric neurology practice at Harvard didn't fit what I had been taught. Two, my research yielded insights I could never have expected. And three, I lucked out in terms of timing. My rethinking of autism coincided with an explosion of science on so many different levels.

This book has been informed by entirely new fields with names like epigenetics, systems biology, gut microbiology, nutrigenomics, and metabolomics, as well as by new revelations in neuroscience, gastroenterology, environmental science, and immunology. We have new tools that allow us to screen tens of thousands of genes in less time than it used to take us to find one. We can now examine single neurons or watch how clumps of them interact. We can explore how the balance of microbes in people's guts changes their health and their brains. New technologies and new research have uncovered previously hidden interconnections, allowing us to frame autism in a way that simply wasn't possible even five years ago.

But this is fundamentally not a science book. It is a book of success stories that make sense biologically.

I believe these triumphs have huge implications for medicine and science and the way we think about autism—and perhaps for much more. I believe it is so dramatic that it calls for a revolution in how we think and what we do.

MARTHA HERBERT, MD, PHD

PART I

Take a Fresh Look at Autism

CHAPTER 1

Go for the Extraordinary

Caleb tore himself away from a game with his sisters, bounced into the kitchen, and asked his mom what she was making for dinner. It was one of his favorites: gluten-free pasta and ground beef.

He started to turn back to the girls, but paused. "Mom," he said, as casually as if he were commenting on the weather, "my autism is gone."

"How do you know?" his astonished mother managed to ask.

"It's easy to be with people now," the ten-year-old said matter-of-factly, and then headed back to his younger sisters.

Joy Petersen* stared, dumbfounded for a few seconds in the middle of the kitchen. It wasn't until two months later that she realized he was right.

Caleb has his father's bright blue eyes, his mother's dark hair, and a complexion that reflects his mixed Dominican American heritage. He is still looking up at five feet, and his voice remains a little boy's for now. He wants to be a zoologist when he grows up, and is already talking about going away to college, although he understands that his parents will be sad to see him go.

Joy recently took him to a new doctor, a specialist in treating children with autism and other special needs. Caleb noticed the photographs

---

* All names of individuals who are not experts have been changed, except in the case of Judy Endow, who is an expert as well as an individual with autism.

covering the doctor's wall and asked why the doctor was holding a gun in one of them. After talking to Caleb and his parents for a while, the doctor announced that Caleb didn't fit the criteria for autism anymore. "Yeah!" Caleb said, jumping up and pumping his arms. His mother began to sob uncontrollably.

Joy used to dream of the day someone would say her son was no longer autistic. Of the day he'd come up to her, say he loved her, and really mean it.

That day was unimaginable when Caleb was four, still had no language, and was so afraid that he would wail and cry when anyone other than his parents came within five feet. Joy said she would put her fingertips on his body and he would scream as if somebody had hit him. Taking care of Caleb was so overwhelming that she would often find herself in tears. There were times when she was so afraid of hurting him in her anger and stress, that she'd put him down, walk into her bedroom, shut herself in her closet, and collapse on the floor, crying.

The doctors and therapists told her she had to be realistic. Your son will probably be like this forever, they said. You can try lots of different things, but none has been proven to work.

Joy decided to start trying them anyway. And to her surprise, everything seemed to work, at least a little. No one thing took the autism away, she said, but all of it put together helped a lot.

By the time Caleb was in first grade, everyone thought she'd succeeded. He was able to follow simple instructions. His repetitive behaviors—the spinning, stick tapping, and high-pitched noises—had mostly stopped. He was able to sit in a mainstream classroom with an aide. This is as good as he's going to get, they told Joy. You've done the best you can.

But she wasn't satisfied. Her heart told her that there was more to do.

"I still had a disconnected boy," she said.

"People would tell me he's high functioning, he follows directions—and I'm like that's not what I want . . . I want a boy I can look in the eye and tell him I love him, and he knows what I'm saying . . . I want a boy who can look *me* in the eye and tell me he loves me . . . I want a boy who can take in the world and absorb it, not run away from it . . . Absorb it, not run away from it," she repeats for emphasis.

She has that boy now.

See What We Believe or Believe What We See

For decades, most doctors told parents that autism was a genetic problem in their child's brain, and that it wasn't going anywhere—that they should expect their toddler's troubles would be with him/her forever. Autism had long been defined by its deficits, by what the child is believed unable to do: communicate, control himself, function like everyone else. Parents might make improvements around the edges—reduce the tantrums, limit the crazy behaviors, get the child to follow directions—but the essential deficits would remain.

After years of researching autism and treating patients at Massachusetts General Hospital, after years of meeting children like Caleb, I have come to the conclusion that the views I had been taught simply couldn't be right.

I have met many, many people like Caleb who are doing remarkably well, often after making improvements more dramatic than anyone ever dreamed possible. Some showed amazing bursts of improvement, transforming from nonverbal and withdrawn to A-student with lots of friends. Some reached adulthood with a stable job and just a few quirks. Some still can't talk but communicate through painting, music, eloquent words typed on a keyboard, or glassblowing. Some, now adults, are professionals, parents, artists, friends, or all of the above.

It may be difficult to imagine now, as you are struggling to help a four-year-old who screams more than he speaks, but many people with autism have grown up to lead fulfilling, productive lives.

The more I worked with my patients, the more I realized I had a choice: to "see what I believed" or to "believe what I see." If I believed that autism was a genetically determined, lifelong brain impairment, then I would have to deny to myself the extraordinary capabilities and changes I saw in my patients. If I believed what I saw, then I would have to rethink everything I knew about autism.

That's what I proceeded to do, and you are reading the result of that exploration.

For going on a decade and a half, I have thrown myself into taking a fresh look at autism. I have probed into generations of science and compared the research with the theories built around this evidence. I have been inspired by a growing body of exciting new findings and new areas of research, which point to new ways of helping people with autism. And I have allowed myself to be touched by people with autism who offered me fresh perspectives and ideas and expanded my world.

More than Genes and Brain: Also Whole Body and Environment

In all my research and reading, I have never found proof of the genes-hopelessly-mess-up-the-brain-for-life model of autism. Genes absolutely affect the brain, but there's no solid proof that they're the only players.

Geneticists have been searching for autism's "smoking gun" for more than a decade. But though more discoveries are on the way, so far they have identified genetic "defects" in only a small minority of people with autism—leaving the vast majority of cases of autism genetically unexplained.

Meanwhile, babies who seem normal for the first year or two regress into autism. Scientists used to believe that all autism was caused by brain damage before birth. Some children with autism do seem different from the start. But a lot of children appear perfectly fine before slipping away over weeks or months. Studies of home videos and direct observations have confirmed that this occurs. Regression into autism makes it hard to just blame genes that kick in late, and makes you wonder about whether environmental stressors play a role, too.

And many children do get better. There is no proof behind the common assumption that if the diagnosis involves a genetic mutation—such as fragile X or idic(15), or others presumed present but not found yet—the person is totally frozen with "impairment" and "deficits" for life. In 2008 I was among a group of researchers who published an article called "Can children with autism recover? If so, how?" Some of these researchers had shown that between 3 and 25 percent of children once diagnosed with autism are eventually told they do not have the condition. How could this happen? Their genes certainly don't change in a few years, so they were either misdiagnosed or, as in the case of Caleb—who was rigorously diagnosed—after lots of treatment, their symptoms faded so much that they no longer belong on the autism spectrum. Many others who don't "recover" still greatly improve.

Autism can even change over minutes, hours, or days—and then change back. Children with fever or on steroids for a medical problem like asthma can show improvements in communication and social interaction, which fade after the fever goes away or the steroids are stopped. If autism were totally genetically hardwired this couldn't happen.

Moreover, genetics cannot explain the rising frequency of the condition. When I first got involved in autism research in 1995, people thought that 1 out of every 3,300 children had autism. As I write, the figure is approaching 1 in 100. Genes take generations to evolve, so either we have been oblivious to autism, or something other than genetics is causing autism more often. There is still some debate about whether autism is truly rising or whether factors like greater awareness and diagnosing people we would have missed in the past are causing at least part of the increase.

By now, most researchers agree that genes usually don't act on their own to cause autism. Genes may lead to vulnerability—they may "load the gun"—but so much of the time, it's environment that "pulls the trigger."

Finally, although I'm a Harvard neurologist—an expert in the brain and nervous system—I have come to believe that just as autism is not simply a genetics problem, it is not simply a brain problem, either. Autism involves the whole body. As a physician, I've seen so many autistic children with similar medical problems that I can't believe it's just a coincidence. And we know through thousands of scientific papers and an ocean of clinical experience that the health of the body can affect the function of the brain.

At this point, I think there is enough evidence to say that while autism certainly involves the brain, it is really a problem of the whole body, including the brain, from molecules to cells, from organs to metabolism, from immune to digestive systems. Even for those with autism who show no obvious medical problems, take a careful look for hidden issues.

An Autism Revolution

If you add environment to genes, add body to brain, take seriously the powerful brilliance of many people with autism and the profound transformations and loss of diagnoses we are seeing more and more, you get a very different story than the hopeless-genetic-lifelong-brain-damage tale that most of us thought was the truth.

The story you get is of problems that can be solved and extraordinary capabilities that can come out of hiding and make powerful impacts on the world.

Caleb got better, in part, because his mother was persistent and she believed in his full potential even when everyone told her he had improved enough. If he could really get better, how many other kids can get better, too? How many others have hidden brilliance that the world needs to see? How many more can feel happier and more comfortable? My commitment is to transform autism so everyone gets their best shot at becoming all they can be. I know so many children like Caleb and so many brilliant and fulfilled people with autism that I feel ethically obliged to tell these stories so we can figure out what makes them possible. Armed with this knowledge, we can go forward and make this great opportunity accessible to as many people as we can. Your child may not be able to make the transformation that Caleb has—their kind of autism may work differently or need another kind of approach. But right now we can't tell who can broaden their options and who can't, so we should hold out the possibility of real, meaningful quality-of-life improvements for everyone.

Journey to the Revolution

How did I get from the genes-broke-the-brain approach to the whole-body, transformative approach that I am giving you now? Through my patients, and through my science.

My Patients

When I finished my neurology training in the mid-1990s, I started doing research, and I began seeing lots of children with learning and behavioral problems. In my clinic, I thought my job as a pediatric neurologist was to see if I could find underlying medical reasons for the difficulties the children were having. I was taught to run genetic tests, to look for seizures and "inborn errors of metabolism"—serious, known diseases of the body's electrical and chemical systems. I dutifully ran all the required tests, and 9 times out of 10, I didn't find anything diagnosable. But that didn't mean that everyone who tested normally on these tests was fine—far from it. Instead I kept noticing that many of my patients weren't feeling well. Some of them experienced frequent infections, some had diarrhea, some couldn't sleep, some had rashes, and lots had allergies. Many had all of the above. A lot had all kinds of additional problems that didn't necessarily fit their diagnosis and a troublingly large number came in with whole strings of diagnoses, as well as a long list of specialists they were seeing and boatloads of medications.

I began asking my patients more medical questions—not just about the brain but about everything I could think of. I also started realizing that these patients needed help with their whole-body problems, not just with their behavior and learning problems. It dawned on me that while I had been trained to look for rare genetic and metabolic conditions, most of my patients were suffering from much more common problems that were being overlooked by pediatricians and other specialists.

What kept frustrating me with my patients was that their problems often didn't meet the criteria for any diagnosable disease. They seemed to be in a "gray zone"—in a no-man's-land between solidly healthy and clearly diseased. The EEG test I used to examine their brain waves would have unusual electrical spikes and rhythms that seemed to indicate a problem, but since there was no evidence of seizures their test results usually read "probably normal." Their metabolic studies would show abnormal levels of chemicals and nutrients, but the official report would read "abnormalities do not fit any known pattern. Normal study." A colonoscopy might show signs of inflammation, but not enough to meet criteria for ulcerative colitis or Crohn's disease. And without a clear diagnosis, there was no standard treatment to prescribe. Some parents told me that as toddlers their children were unable to sleep more than two hours at a time, bounced off the walls all day long, and had frequent diarrhea so acidic that it would blister their skin and burn through the couch cushions. But so often they were told "this is a stage; your child will grow out of it."

As this played out over and over again, I kept thinking of the story about the doctor who tells the patient, "There is nothing wrong with you. But on the other hand, there is nothing right with you, either."

My Science

I started out studying MRI brain scans from children with autism and with language problems. I was studying anatomy—the structure of the brain. My original goal was to find the specific areas of the brain that were causing the defining hallmarks of autism—communication difficulties, social problems, and unusual behaviors—to help the geneticists and biologists find out what caused this and what we could do. However, as hard as I looked, I didn't find broken brain regions. Instead I found, as did others, that the whole brain was larger—that there was something different about its cable networks. How could a large brain or cable network issues have anything to do with an autism spectrum condition defined by specific behaviors?

What I found was that brains were larger in these school-age children because of enlargement of "white matter"—the cable system that connects neurons near and far so the brain can think. This meant that instead of there being a few hubs with problems, the whole brain network was different. At the same time, other researchers were studying how the brain functions. They started finding that it wasn't the activity of a few little areas that was different. Instead the connections across large areas seemed weaker—not a lot weaker in any one place, but a little weaker all over. The psychologist Marcel Just of Carnegie Mellon University calls this "underconnectivity"—another network problem.

If brain networks are weaker, the kinds of thinking that require pulling lots of information together all at the same time will suffer. And come to think of it, the areas of weakness that define autism—communication, social interaction, and behavioral flexibility—all involve a whole lot of brain coordination. I began to realize that autism wasn't about something in any one place being broken—it was about network problems.

Finally, in 2005, a research team at Johns Hopkins led by Carlos Pardo reported finding inflammation in the brain tissue of people with autism. So this wasn't just about a wiring diagram—it was about cells and their health. I started wondering if the bigger brain size had to do with inflammation. Other researchers were finding related immune problems in blood tests. And I was seeing possibly related medical problems in my patients. Maybe the whole body, including the brain, was having one big health and network problem.

All of this started to connect up in my mind. All these problems seemed to be networked together like a big web.

Brain networks are built out of brain cells. The brain cells are in the body and the whole body is having health problems.

If the brain cells are having health problems, too, wouldn't that cut into how well they can do their jobs? So maybe the brain networks in autism are weaker because the cells are having a tough time.

If that's the case, then improving the whole body's health might trickle up to the brain and put more energy into the brain networks. With more energetic networks, the brain should have more resources to coordinate thinking, feeling, sensation, body movement, regulation of body functions— all the things that are challenged for people with autism.

RESEARCH SPOTLIGHT: EXPANDING THE BRAIN'S WEB

Most of the research on brain problems of people with autism simply describes how their brains are different from those of people without autism, and how they work less well. Many dozens of researchers have shown that the brain's web is usually less well "networked" in people with autism than in their non-autistic peers. Most of those researchers seem to assume that problems in connectivity are hardwired into the brain, due to genetic mutations.

David Beversdorf, a pediatric neurologist and brain imaging researcher at the University of Missouri, wondered instead if these problems were changeable, if the connectivity could be improved. He tested a medication called propranolol, a blood pressure drug also used for anxiety and stage fright, to see if it would improve brain connectivity—and it did! Minutes after taking the propranolol, the brains of people with autism expanded their connectivity networks. While this study did not test whether propranolol is safe or effective as a treatment for autism, Beversdorf did discover something vitally important about how the brain in autism works. The connectivity problems are not hardwired. They can change, and fast. Stress creates noise and chaos, so the signals are drowned out. Reduce the noise and chaos, and the brain will increase its bandwidth and access its networks more fully.

How Does Autism Happen?

No one yet knows, and we may never know for certain what causes autism. Some people want to blame rising autism rates on our modern environment, filled with potential toxins, new germs, and stress. I think these play an important role, and not just for autism—after all, allergies, immune problems, and many chronic diseases are on the rise, too. But if there were a single, clear trigger for autism, we would have already found it. There may be many kinds of autism, most with lots of different triggers.

My observations and hundreds of stories I've heard lead me to believe that what we see as autism often emerges or worsens after a series of challenges to a young body and brain. These might include environmental factors like air pollution, viruses, or something that happened to our grandparents; they might be the food we eat, the water we drink, or the stresses of daily life. Or maybe all those things together. For some reason, which we may never fully understand, in some young children all these strains and burdens of everyday life get too heavy. Instead of bouncing back from the pressure, these young bodies are pushed over an edge.

Many of the insults may be very slight, invisible even. A child becomes vulnerable, perhaps from a difficult delivery that leaves restrictions on sucking or moving; or from an infection during pregnancy that makes the baby more prone to infection; or an inherited risk for immune problems.

In most children, such events mean nothing—the infection clears quickly, the muscle pain is short-lived, and the baby's natural resilience kicks in.

But sometimes these challenges are compounded by others. Maybe the infant is exposed to a toxin that weakens his liver, a course of antibiotics knocks down the good bacteria in her gut, continuing muscle tightness makes the baby reluctant to explore the world. At each step of the way, the systems of the body are prevented from flourishing, and the brain is distracted by physical problems from exploring the wondrous world.

And at some point, the *total load* of these problems reaches a tipping point. Now one and a half or two or three or four years old, the child's body and brain have been battered so much by the world that they have lost the resources to protect themselves. The body can no longer support the brain's full range of capabilities, and in order to conserve itself the brain pulls back from making sense of the world. Under these circumstances the child turns in on himself for protection against a painful, overwhelming world—because it's the best he or she can do. We look at the child from the outside and see a "regression." We can't see inside the child's body or brain but from the outside we see strange behaviors, and we call it "autism."

Caleb fits this pattern, as do the others whose stories I will tell you.

His mother's first child, Caleb got stuck on the way out. He was trapped for two hours as Joy's labor stalled, and his head ended up misshapen and squashed. Caleb recovered quickly (though part of his head remained flat for years) and he seemed to be a totally typical baby. But he was sick a lot. By age two, Caleb had had thirteen ear infections, each one treated by ever stronger antibiotics. His mother noticed that he had an unusually large head, wearing an adult-sized hat by the age of three, but the pediatrician told Joy not to worry. Caleb was perfectly healthy, the doctor said.

When Caleb was about sixteen months old, he stopped speaking. He became fearful and anxious. He'd flap his arms anytime anyone even looked like they were coming near him. Joy took him back to the pediatrician, but the doctor wasn't worried. The boy was normal; the only problem was Joy's anxiety, the doctor said.

Joy brought him back again at twenty months, and again at twenty-three months. This time she told her doctor she wasn't leaving without a referral to a specialist. Caleb was sent to see a speech pathologist. At the first appointment, the pathologist told Joy she was pretty sure the boy had autism, and sent him for further testing that confirmed the diagnosis.

Somehow, these seemingly insignificant events had piled up into a dramatic problem.

From Parts to Whole

After Caleb was diagnosed, he started getting behavioral therapies, but his progress was very slow. Joy got frustrated with this and sought out other alternatives. He started making more progress with both sensory and auditory integration training. Real breakthroughs occurred when Joy started addressing his body problems. As this progress consolidated, he was able to get more benefit from behavioral and relational therapies. Just as many things had contributed to his getting worse, many things contributed to his getting better.

From a whole-body, whole-system perspective, autism's behaviors are important, but they are just one part of the interconnected web that is autism. To help your child get better, you need to recognize *all* these parts, and look for ways of addressing them.

In this book I will walk you through the major parts of the web, chapter by chapter. Here are the parts of the web and the problems Caleb showed at each part when he was four or five years old:

Genes and environment: No problem genes were identified, but he had trouble with infection and, as he later learned, with some of the foods he ate regularly. His environment also included a very devoted family determined to help him.

Cell problems: His cholesterol was found to be too low; lab tests after his diagnosis showed he had low levels of antioxidants and was deficient in fatty acids. By the end of the school day, he was totally wiped out.

Body health problems: Caleb had constant ear infections for his first few years, and his tonsils were always swollen, suggesting a continuing infection. He had gut infections, frequent urination, lots of tummy aches, diarrhea, and irregular bowel movements, and according to his doctor he wasn't gaining enough weight. He always had deep, dark circles under his eyes.

Brain health problems: Caleb had an unusually large head, and the right back side of his skull remained flat after a difficult birth. He was often foggy and disoriented.

Brain processing problems: He couldn't stand to be touched. He flapped his arms, tapped sticks, and spun in circles repeatedly. He constantly made high-pitched noises or screamed for apparently no reason. He had frequent meltdowns, had food cravings and his sleep was shallow and fitful.

Thinking, feeling, attending problems: He couldn't follow simple directions. Instead of asking him to take off his jacket, Joy would have to break the task down into its smallest parts—first, grab your left sleeve with your right arm and pull—before Caleb could follow. He was inattentive, hyperactive, anxious, and rigid. Everything had to be done his way and the same way every time.

Communicating and relating problems: Caleb was disconnected and withdrawn from others. He wouldn't make eye contact. He laughed at inappropriate times. He didn't speak.

Blockages to creativity and transcendence: He couldn't draw a picture, and he couldn't express himself to others.

Is any of this familiar to you?

This is not who your child "is"—it's who they *became.*

When you look at your child being so challenging and difficult it may be hard to believe that there isn't something fundamentally and permanently wrong. But please take a fresh look at your child. Think about the snowball effect that Caleb went through in his first two years before he "regressed" into autism. It was a process that happened. It wasn't destiny. There were many factors that contributed to his problems, and I believe there are many parts of this process that can be reversed. Joy unwound Caleb's autism by hunting relentlessly for specific problems that could be addressed. You can learn to do this, too.

Your child became this way over time due to some kind of cascade effect that likely included both genes and environment, creating an ever more complicated web of problems. Once your child is tangled in this web, it may seem like there's nothing you can do to make a major difference. But the stories of thousands of people with autism who have gotten healthier suggest there is plenty you can do to change the course of your child's life.

In each chapter of this book I suggest ways you can help untangle the threads of this web, removing obstacles and shoring up your child's natural resilience.

Chapter 2 will show you how *genes and environment* set the stage for your child's particular brand of autism, and how you can identify challenges and build up strengths.

Chapter 3 will tell you about how to build *cell health* to support a healthy body and brain.

Chapter 4 will show you how to build *whole-body health* by supporting the digestive and immune systems.

Chapter 5 explains how to build the ***brain's physical health,*** which lays the foundation for the brain to function fluidly and efficiently.

Chapter 6 will help you identify and remove obstacles to achieving the ***best possible brain sensitivity, coordination, and function.***

Chapter 7 will help you ***take a whole-body approach to day-to-day problems*** with behaving, thinking, feeling, focusing, learning, communicating, and relating.

Chapter 8 will give you a taste of how good life can get when it all comes together, when the pain has faded and your child can ***celebrate his or her unique gifts.***

Chapter 9 will show you how to put these suggestions all together and ***track your progress*** as well as ***pool your data*** so you can help other families in addition to your own.

Chapter 10 will help you get your own life in order so you can create the ***best possible environment for your family and your next child,*** stopping the cascade before it begins.

Remember: The web is interconnected. Tug one thread and you can affect the rest of the web. Troubles in one part of it make life harder for all the other parts. Restoring health in some areas makes it easier for other areas to do better, too. For example, treating the gut sometimes helps the brain work better. And helping the brain work better sometimes calms the gut.

I hope you'll come with me on this journey toward health and resilience. I have watched so many people with autism become incredibly creative, extraordinary children, teenagers, and adults that it has made me greedy for more. I want to see everyone else's autistic child have the same chance.

A WEB OF PROBLEMS

Our whole-body, whole-brain webs are constantly sending signals at every imaginable level—inside our cells, among our cells, using molecules and electricity, in little packets, and in complicated waves and patterns. When we're healthy, vibrant, and creative, these signals travel clearly and strongly from one part of the web to another.

When we're sick, stuck, or have low energy, the parts of the web don't work well, and they are not well connected, either. Our cells, our organs, our brain can drag and so our performance drags.

- When the **body's web** is strained you get body problems—allergies, clumsiness, digestive problems, and more.
- When the **brain's web** is strained you get confusion and overload. The signals get drowned out by static noise and the coordination of the brain starts to fall apart. We can't see the brain confusion directly, but we do see the behaviors it creates. In autism, this brain confusion looks from the outside like "deficits in communication, social interaction, and behavior"—pretty much the accepted definition of autism.

Think of it like an orchestra. An orchestra is the sum of its parts, and all the parts need to be synchronized and in harmony. With strong musicians, high-quality, well-tuned instruments, and a good conductor, an orchestra makes magnificent music. With out-of-tune instruments, musicians who are not feeling well, and a distracted conductor, an orchestra sounds jarring and dissonant. To make the orchestra sound better you need to repair the parts that have problems, so harmony and synchrony can be restored.

I Know My Child Is "in There"

What happens to someone who is diagnosed with autism after a deterioration like Caleb's, or a process that may have begun even earlier? Do they disappear forever? I don't think there's proof that this has to be true. Many parents talk about seeing flashes of their "real" child trapped inside the autism. The autism they describe—and that I have seen in my patients—is not a monotonous life sentence. It changes from day to day—even moment to moment. The potential for a functional brain seems "in there." A largely nonverbal child will burst out with a fully articulate sentence during a time of joy or crisis. A fifty-year-old autistic man will get help with a previously undiagnosed hearing problem, learn to keyboard, and have the first conversation of his life with his eighty-year-old mother.

The brain seems to be working and taking in the world even when a casual glance at the person offers the opposite impression. I've heard of plenty of examples of five-year-olds, autistic and remote since age two, who "pop out" at such a high level after intensive treatment that it's clear they were there all along.

Parents of recovered children are often embarrassed when their child recalls in exquisite detail events from when they were deeply autistic and their parents thought they were totally oblivious.

Recently, Caleb apologized to his mom for being a "monster" when he was little, screaming all the time and driving her crazy. Then, he told her, "there's still something wrong with me. I don't know what or why."

We don't know if Caleb's autistic traits are gone or whether he has learned to compensate for them. Joy is taking Caleb in for more testing now to see if there's more that can be done to improve his focus and his organizational skills. He still feels a bit chaotic and disorganized, she said.

Knowing your child is "in there" may be part of your own powerful motivation to read this book and do everything you can for your child, as it was for Joy. I will explain to you much more in the chapters to come and symptomswhy you should believe what you see. It should help you to understand that your child's brain is not broken or impaired but challenged, overwhelmed, and obstructed.

MY FIRST SUCCESS

When I tried using this web-based approach with my patients, instead of prescribing a series of unrelated drugs, each targeted at one of their many di- agnoses and symptoms, I started working to make their whole web stronger. I aimed to correct the little dysfunctions where there were low-risk relevant things that I could do.

A nine-year-old patient taught me that these small changes can make a dramatic difference. She had had reflux from the time she was an infant, in- numerable infections, and countless courses of antibiotics every year. She was labeled bipolar and had asthma, nasty diarrhea, and fainting spells. She also had bumpy skin on the backs of her arms and on her face. Since I knew those bumps could be a sign of essential fatty acid deficiency, I cautiously started her on fish oil. I also put her on probiotics to help with the diarrhea. I expected some small improvements.

Instead, within a month, almost all of the girl's problems vanished. Her anxiety, reflux, asthma, and diarrhea greatly diminished, and she was able to stop nearly all of her medications. My treatments didn't just fix isolated symptoms—they helped her whole system. With that little assist, her basic web was able to snap back to a healthy shape, and at a rate far faster than Caleb's later. Maybe I was just lucky, and I never thought this was a quick fix for bipolar disorder, but even so I was also hooked. If an intervention so simple could have such a broad impact, how could I do this for more people?

Build the Revolution by Helping Your Child

This whole-body, web view of autism remains a work in progress. The stories impel us to do much more research. If we can learn how Caleb and others climb out of autism's limitations, we may get closer to knowing how they got into trouble in the first place. This science of recovery will shine a huge spotlight that illuminates much more than autism itself.

But meanwhile, your child needs help now. I am presenting you with a plausible, safe, and rational approach that you can follow while we wait for the science to mature. I don't have incontrovertible proof that the ideas in this book will work for your child. What I have instead, what I will offer you here, is a framework of commonsense, straightforward strategies that have made a profound difference in the lives of children like Caleb. It transforms autism from a blanket life sentence to a set of more specific problems that can be addressed systematically. I can't promise you the same fantastic outcome he got; I can't promise that your child will walk off the autism spectrum in ten easy steps.

But I can promise you that if you follow this whole-body method, you will gain new insights into your child, new ways to approach autism, and new hope for the extraordinary potential of each autistic child—not just to be "special," but to make a meaningful contribution to their community and their world. You are likely to see real and hopefully major tangible improvements in your child's quality of life—and yours as well. Many parents before you have found creative ways to manage these challenges.

The strength of this view is that it is fundamentally filled with hope. Just as autism may emerge after an accumulation of seemingly minor insults, so too may little changes have a major impact in rolling it back. Most of the people I'll introduce you to in this book experienced profound transformations, but they didn't do radical things. They changed what they ate. They took vitamin supplements and got exercise and did different types of sensory and movement therapies. Their parents learned how to join them in their world and let them find ways back that worked for them. They got help from doctors and therapists. But the underlying foundation was supporting the whole web—and persisting and taking charge.

We Can't Afford Not to Have an Autism Revolution

It's terrifying to imagine our future without this revolution.

The financial costs alone of raising our autistic children are staggering, with estimates ranging from $35 billion to $90 billion per year just in the United States. That assumes autism rates stop increasing, which hasn't happened yet. And of course, children with autism usually grow into adults with autism, so those costs will be with us for decades if we don't take action. At a time when America is still reeling from recession and when budget cutting seems to be the nation's top priority, what will we do if there is not enough to go around to give everyone the help they need? Wouldn't it be a good idea to address autism early and effectively?

If we continue to believe that autism is a lifelong, hopeless condition we will be patient with slow progress because we won't see how you might fundamentally help people. When we see people with autism improving, we will deny that they had autism to begin with. This kind of circular thinking breeds inertia, countless missed opportunities, and lost dreams, all of which damages not just the individuals who are left behind but the fabric of our whole society. More and more people will be autistic, more hearts broken, and more communities financially stressed.

Now take a moment to envision a world where everyone believes that there are many parts of autism we can do something about, and that when people with autism are transformed, it is real and has something vital to teach us. Think about the energy and resources we would pour into tackling solvable problems. Imagine all the loving and happy family interactions, the creative brilliance unleashed, and the benefit to all society.

Thousands of children like Caleb are teaching us the paths to success. They do it in spite of a system that tells them they can't, and shouldn't. Imagine what we could do if we took these successes seriously and learned how to achieve them better and for many more people.

I believe that autism is not a genetic tragedy, but rather an unfolding and unprecedented challenge related to many other health and environmental crises. We need to build a world that makes us healthy.

Remember that for your child you are a pathbreaker. You may become a pathbreaker for others as well. The first step is perhaps the most potent: Take a stand with hope that your child can change, not just a little bit, but profoundly. Joy stayed firm with the vision that her son could get the most out of life. You can do this, too.

Caleb got a lot better, many other children get a lot better, and your child may, too. Most children can achieve at least some improvements. These experiences can teach others how to become healthy, move beyond autism, and fulfill their potential to be extraordinary.

WHAT YOU CAN DO

See Your Web, Build Your Vision

I suggest you begin the healing process by taking a fresh look at the autism in your life. If you haven't already, get a notebook to log your journey.

Now take a metaphorical step back from the struggle you had getting out of the house this morning, last weekend's epic temper tantrum, and your last visit to the doctor—and begin to envision your child's own unique web, thread by thread. I recommend that parents begin by making a list similar to the one I made for Caleb, but including strengths as well as problems. You can use the list below as a resource. Add things not on the list as well. If you're a visual person, you can design your own web. You may want to get fancy, using colors and different thicknesses of lines to indicate the size of the problem or magnitude of strength. If you're not, you can make columns and then group strengths and challenges under categories.

Or simply checking off the items below that seem relevant to your life may help you gain a new perspective.

When you're done, take a minute to survey your own personal autism web for the first time.

Characteristics and Symptoms
- Incredible depth of knowledge in one subject
- Ability to recognize patterns
- Often has diarrhea/constipation
- Sometimes has difficulty sleeping
- Sometimes seems tuned in to the world, sometimes not
- Can seem extremely frustrated, particularly by an inability to communicate
- Knows more than they can show
- Loves solving puzzles
- Sometimes aggressive/sometimes not
- Seems overwhelmed in busy places
- Has strong food preferences
- Prefers certain textures of food over others
- Sometimes extremely lacking in energy
- Gets sick often
- Has seizures
- Has poor muscle tone
- Is happy a lot of the time
- Seems content within him/herself
- Loves taking apart machines
- Has trouble making eye contact
- Can't listen and make eye contact at the same time
- Unable or unwilling to develop friendships
- Doesn't show, bring, or point out objects of interest to others
- Doesn't need approval from others to pursue an interest or passion
- Prefers to play alone
- Has meltdowns

- Speech is delayed, difficult, or not present at all
- Mathematical ability far exceeds communication skills
- Unable or unwilling to sustain or initiate a conversation
- Uses language idiosyncratically—repeats dialogue from movies and TV, speaks in nonsense words, or constructs nontraditional sentences
- Doesn't play make-believe games
- Sets toys up or lines them up but does not play with them
- Seems more interested in play with parts of toys, such as wheels that spin, than with the whole
- Gets overwhelmed by a change in routine
- Takes pleasure in rituals and/or repetitive actions
- Behavior improves when feverish, on antibiotics, while fasting, or from some other unusual trigger
- Frequently seems frightened
- Interprets instructions and metaphors very literally
- Enjoys repetitive physical mannerisms, such as flapping or twisting
- Loves spinning on a swing or swivel chair
- Gets caught up in parts of objects rather than the whole
- Is extremely sensitive—needs deep pressure or frequent hugs or hates to be touched
- Covers eyes or ears constantly
- Please list other strengths and challenges you believe are related to your/your child's autism: _____
- _____
- _____
- _____

Now take a moment to close your eyes and envision what you want for your child. Make it really concrete. Then write it down.

_____

_____

_____

_____

_____

_____

You can do this next exercise now, regularly, and whenever life gets particularly tough:

a. Visualize or imagine how your child is now and take a minute to explore what it's like. Use the web diagram you just made to help you. Whatever comes up in your mind is fine, including feelings of grief, disappointment, anger, or blame. Just note them.

b. Then visualize what you want for your child and take a minute to explore what it's like. Focus on the parts that are the most meaningful and give you the most satisfaction.

c. Now imagine these two images merging together. Imagine pathways growing from the present situation to the vision you want. Though you may not know what they are yet, there are many ways to get from the present situation to your vision. Aim to find them.

d. Remind yourself that there is much more to your child than what you can see right now.

e. It may be hard to feel genuine gratitude when you start on this path or when your child has just spread his own feces all over the walls. But notice the good moments when they come, so you can learn to hang on to them if things get bad. Over time, you may come to see your child as a teacher who will bring out how extraordinary you are, and see too how much you can do when faced with an extraordinary challenge.

In the next chapter, I will explain how genes and environment work together, and offer suggestions for making the most of what you've got.

KEEP IN MIND

- Autism is a collection of problems that can be addressed, and many of those can be solved.
- Autism emerges from a cascade of problems, and with careful and persistent effort many parts of this cascade may be reversed.

- Every gain matters.
- Most of the problems of autism are not unique to autism.

But also remember
- No single problem causes autism by itself.
- No single treatment fixes autism by itself.
- You are not to blame for your child's autism or lack of progress. But you may be able to help your child do better by building up health and resilience, and by removing impediments.

CHAPTER 2

Know What You Can't Control—
and What You Can

I f you're convinced that brain conditions are lifelong and irreversible, consider this story about a Norwegian mother of two: In January 1934, Borgny Egeland was watching her infant son Dag, born healthy, descend into the same kind of mental retardation that had already claimed her daughter Liv. Looking for answers, Egeland sought out Dr. Ivar Asbjørn Følling, a Norwegian nutrition expert, who agreed to investigate. Her children, she told Følling, had a funny "mousy" odor, and when he used a simple chemical test for diabetes, their urine turned green instead of the expected brownish purple. After several months of research, Følling deduced that the children's urine contained a substance called phenylpyruvic acid, which had never before been noted in human urine. He then collected samples from 430 patients at area mental hospitals and discovered that eight of them also excreted phenylpyruvic acid in their urine. All eight were considered mentally retarded and most, like the woman's children, had light hair and skin, broad shoulders, stooping posture, and an awkward gait.

He concluded that their metabolic problem was hereditary. There were three pairs of siblings among the ten. In three families the parents were closely related, and two of those parents had children from second marriages who were unaffected by retardation. Følling decided that the disorder must be passed on from healthy parents who were unknowing carriers; both had to have the genetic fluke for the children to inherit the problem.

Følling also figured out that the ten had a metabolic blockage. Their bodies could not transform one amino acid (phenylalanine, found in high-protein foods) into another, tyrosine. Tyrosine is needed to make the neurotransmitters dopamine and adrenaline, which affect mood and anxiety, and the pigment melanin (hence their pale complexions), among other things. And without the ability to change into tyrosine, phenylalanine was piling up and turning into a toxic substance called phenylpyruvate. Infants with this disorder, later named phenylketon-uria, or PKU, were born seemingly healthy, but quickly became disabled. The protein in their food triggered a buildup of toxic phenylpyruvate, causing retardation, autistic symptoms, and a host of other problems.

The Future Is Not Foretold

Today, in most countries, newborn screening of every baby includes a test for phenylpyruvic acid and children found to have high levels are immediately placed on an extremely low-protein diet supplemented by tyrosine, which they can't make themselves. This dietary change, though cumbersome, completely prevents the disabling symptoms of PKU and allows them to lead full, "normal" lives.

PKU is not reversible; the buildup of phenylalanine irrevocably dam-ages cells in the brain and body. But it's preventable if the diet is started early enough. And even in adults with PKU, many of whom also have an autism diagnosis, diet matters: Eating an extremely low-protein diet can reduce symptoms such as hyperactivity, depression, anxiety, and psy-chosis, researchers from New York University Medical Center have shown.

So, PKU is a genetic condition triggered by the child's environment, in this case food. It leads otherwise healthy children to develop severe mental and behavioral problems as well as whole-body traits, such as an awkward gait and distinctive coloring. And it is reversible in infancy and treatable later in life, by addressing the same environmental causes that set it in motion in the first place. The genetic vulnerability is still there; the symptoms are not.

In this chapter, I'd like to walk you through research that shows some powerful parallels between PKU and autism. I don't mean to suggest that a dietary change will make a similarly dramatic change in everyone with autism. My point is broader—that autism is similarly affected by the child's environment, and that changes to the environment can have profound effects on the autism.

It's not clear yet how many components of autism are permanent and how many can change or be reversed. But research into two more autism-like conditions also suggests that even when a genetic mutation leads to brain and whole-body problems, the potential for overcoming challenging symptoms remains.

Fragile X Syndrome

In fragile X syndrome, a protein called FMRP is missing because a gene malfunctions. FMRP turns on and off the production of other proteins. Without FMRP, protein production runs amok, like a car whose gas pedal is stuck to the floor. Children born with fragile X have a range of intellectual and physical symptoms. These can include communication problems, hyperactivity, anxiety, moodiness, seizures, gastrointestinal issues, and autistic behaviors. They are often diagnosed with autism as well.

Several researchers and companies are developing drugs that act like a brake on this protein production, unsticking the gas pedal, as it were. If these drugs can normalize the protein production, perhaps some of the symptoms will go away. Though the drugs are still in early stages of development, at the time of this writing, results are encouraging. Mark Bear, the MIT neuroscientist leading this work, says the success with PKU gives him hope that he can do the same for fragile X, and possibly autism as well.

Rett Syndrome

In experiments with adult mice, researchers from the University of Edinburgh turned on the gene that is turned off in Rett syndrome, another condition often associated with autism. The mice, which showed Rett symptoms when the gene was turned off, appeared completely normal after it was turned on—almost as if they'd been given a key they'd been missing all their lives, according to the research. The amazing thing about this research was that it was done in *adult* mice, not young ones, suggesting that the condition is reversible at any age. Neurons don't die in autism, the way they do in Alzheimer's or Lou Gehrig's disease, the researchers noted. So, there's no obvious reason they couldn't be retrained.

"Everyone assumes that autism, schizophrenia, all these things are done deals once the symptoms are there," Adrian Bird, the study's senior author, told *The Boston Globe* in 2007. "But we have to ask ourselves, 'Why do we believe the brain is so fixed and non-plastic?' Maybe we should look more carefully at what else can be reversed."

GENETIC TESTING

Even if genes may not be the only cause of someone's autism, they can still contribute, so it is important to get the best possible information about your child's genetics. New testing technologies now make it feasible to have a much more efficient test at a much lower cost than ever before. The first line of genetic testing, looking for known mutations, is a blood test called chromosomal microarray analysis (CMA). You can get this either from your pediatrician or via referral to a specialist. If the CMA doesn't identify any abnormalities, your doctor may still want to order further specialized genetic tests. There are also tests of your child's metabolism that look for other signs of genetic problems.

Our Understanding of How Genes Work Is Evolving

Scientists used to think that nearly everything about us was contained in our genetic code. Hair color? Set by your DNA. Tendency to be anxious? Again, determined by DNA. Susceptibility to illness? Yup, DNA. But the mapping of the human genome—begun in 1990 and completed in 2003—has changed scientists' understanding of genes. Researchers are increasingly recognizing how much more complex we are than one set of instructions delivered at birth.

The genes that you inherit from your parents do influence your hair color, some of your personality traits, and your likelihood of getting certain diseases. But genes only set the stage. Your genes aren't so much a "blueprint" of who you will become. They are a living document that changes over the course of your life, influenced by the air you breathe, the food you eat, and the experiences and exposures you have. You can't change your (or your child's) underlying genetic code, but you can change many of the inputs those genes receive, avoiding stress and toxins and promoting health.

Genes, we now understand, change over the course of generations, and a single lifetime, through mutation. Genetic mutations aren't always bad—we'd still be bacteria without them. Mutations, essentially, are when a copy of DNA is different from the original. They can come from copying errors in which the units of the DNA—the T, C, G, and A—get duplicated incorrectly, or whole pieces get lost or moved around. When cells make new cells, their DNA must be copied, and sometimes the machinery makes mistakes. Not every car that comes off every assembly line has all the right parts: Some are missing headlights, or cup holders or a single bolt in the wheel well. The factory workers check over the car looking for these mistakes, just as the cell's DNA repair mechanisms seek out and repair most flaws. The errors that don't get caught are mutations. Even if only one mistake slips through for every one billion pairs of amino acids made, there will be three new mistakes every time the DNA is copied.

Mutations can happen during pregnancy, when cells are reproducing rapidly, or as part of aging, when damage accumulates. Many cancers start with genetic mutations, often triggered by environmental exposures like radiation or chemicals. And as men and women age, their sperm and eggs may accumulate genetic abnormalities.

We now know that some children with autism have genetic mutations that their parents don't have. Where did they come from? There is no agreement among scientists about this right now, and studies about such "de novo" mutations are relatively new. But one possibility is that these genetic mutations were triggered by something in the environment.

Some of these new mutations appear to be generated by repetitions or deletions in the genetic code. A parent might have three repetitions of a sequence of T's, C's, G's, or A's, while the child has six—just enough to trigger symptoms, perhaps of autism.

And sometimes genes that aren't a problem for the parent become one for the child, born and raised under different conditions. A driver might never notice a single missing bolt in the car's wheel well. But then a minor fender bender might twist the axle ever so slightly, putting more pressure on the wheel. Over time, the combination of the missing bolt and the added pressure can make for dangerous driving conditions. The same kind of buildup is likely at play in autism.

Scientists have realized in recent years that genes don't even have to be mutated in order to act differently. In many cases, the genes stay the same but their activity changes, with some turning on or off and others up or down. This genetic toggling, called *gene expression,* is a normal activity. All the cells in your body have the same genes, but your brain cells express different genes than your liver cells because they have different jobs to do.

Gene expression changes when the body's needs do. An old person needs different genes activated than a growing child. Gene expression can also be altered by the environment—think of a child who stops growing because of a lack of food; or a cancer triggered by cigarette smoking. These "epigenetic" modifications can even get passed on to the next generation, though the underlying genes stay the same.

The Genetic Side of Autism

Scientists have looked hard for "the" autism gene or small group of genes for a decade—but so far, it's been in vain.

Instead they have found hundreds of genes, each of which accounts for only a small number of people with the diagnosis. There is no "autism gene" anywhere near common enough for a newborn screening test as we have with PKU. Nor do these genes always clearly predict autism. (Just for the record, there are more than five hundred different mutations now associated with PKU, each in its own way—so even single gene disorders can be complicated.)

Before this hunt began, scientists assumed autism would be as genetically driven as PKU or fragile X, because the condition seems to run in families. A family with one child on the spectrum is many times more likely to have a second than would be expected in the general population. And identical twins are more likely to share a diagnosis than fraternal twins, who don't share the same genetic code.

But these family connections don't prove that autism is solely genetic. Not all pairs of identical twins develop autism—and even if they're both on the spectrum, they're often in different places on it. Some genes, like the ones associated with fragile X and Rett syndrome, greatly increase the risk for autism, but not everyone with those conditions develops autism. With fragile X it may be less than half. A recent autism twin study, the largest ever performed, found less shared diagnosis among identical twins and more among fraternal twins than expected, and concluded that environment is more important than heredity in the development of autism.

And for siblings, a common environmental impact could have caused autism in both. After all, they shared the same womb.

RESEARCH SPOTLIGHT: INFLUENCES BEFORE BIRTH

In a 1995 study of identical twins with schizophrenia, researchers found that the odds of both twins having schizophrenia was much higher when they shared a placenta, the pancake-shaped, hormone-producing organ in the womb attached to the umbilical cord. (Identical twins sometimes share a placenta and sometimes get their own.)

Sixty percent of the twin pairs who shared a placenta were both schizophrenic, while only 11 percent of those with different placentas both had the disorder. The researchers said their findings suggest that a mother's viral infection during pregnancy might affect only one placenta, or one more than the other. An infant nurtured in an affected placenta might go on to develop schizophrenia years later, while one in an unaffected placenta might not. Other, more recent research supports this idea that early exposure to viruses plays a role in the development of schizophrenia. It could also be something else.

Clearly then, the uterine environment can make a major difference. And a condition like schizophrenia, long considered genetic, might also have an environmental trigger.

Environment Can Alter a Gene's Importance

The Pima Indians lived for hundreds of years eating food local to their desert environment, and were lean and healthy. When they gave up their native cooking and started eating what's often called an American diet, many of them became obese and diabetic. Does this mean they had a "gene for diabetes"? Or simply that they were eating the wrong foods for their genetic and metabolic makeup?

All of us are walking around with genetic variations that affect us mildly, if at all. We might have a gene that speeds things up. That can be good for handling a problem more efficiently, but it can also make you burn through needed supplies faster. Such mutations may be noticeable only after something else happens to reveal the genetic weakness or strength underneath.

No one has perfect genes. If our environment makes difficult demands on us, and we are not tanked up with good supports, we are all at risk for illness. And we know that children with autism diagnoses are particularly vulnerable; either they're born unhealthy or their health starts to get compromised very early.

To better understand this idea, consider another metaphor:

Imagine a hill at the bottom of a lake. It goes unnoticed for decades or centuries, until a drought hits. As the water level drops, boats start to run aground on it and eventually it's visible above the waterline. A good strong rain can make it disappear again, at least until there's a string of hot days. In the body, environmental influences can raise or lower our metaphorical "water level"—they can fill the lake, so the hill is hidden, or drop the water down, so the risk of boat damage is higher.

Like that pond, your child may have started out perfectly healthy, but the stresses he or she met in the first few months of life uncovered a hidden underlying genetic difficulty: It took an interaction between the terrain and the drought, the genes and the environment, to reveal the problem.

This may be why some parents of children with autism have very mild, autism-like features. Take, for example, an extremely bright but socially awkward parent. He can hold down a job and a conversation, and easily participate in everyday activities; his autistic daughter cannot. Between his generation and the generation of his children, the water level of the lake dropped, exposing more risk, and making traits more extreme.

RARE METABOLIC DISORDERS

A fair number of rare metabolic disorders are often associated with autism. Sometimes genetic mutations break some important link in one of our body's chemical production lines. This can lead to rare but serious problems called "inborn errors of metabolism." Newborns are screened for some of these, including PKU. Other inborn errors of metabolism—often the ones associated with a high risk of autism—don't turn up in the newborn screening or even in standard tests.

There are certain red flags that may cause your doctor to ask for a metabolic workup, looking for one of these errors. Those red flags include: lethargy, having an unusual odor, repeated regression, uncontrolled seizures, extreme developmental delay, being very small for age, having very low muscle tone, deafness, cataracts, certain chronic rashes, or joints that become hard to bend. To get this kind of testing you usually have to go to a specialist.

Some metabolic diseases slow the system down, but they can be treated with extra nutrients to help speed it back up. Others prevent the body from metabolizing or breaking down certain substances; you can prevent harm by withholding those substances, as with PKU. In still others, you will be told situations to avoid—fasting may be a problem, for instance, because your child may not be able to compensate for low blood sugar. For many metabolic disorders, new research may reveal things that can help. The doctor who diagnoses the disorder should be able to tell you what to do.

WHAT YOU CAN DO: FOOD, TOXINS, BUGS, AND STRESS

So, what makes the water in our metaphorical lake drop, revealing the hill? For a lake, hot weather is one environmental stressor. Just as a few days of good soaking rains can make the lake safer for boaters, so many environmental influences can reverse epigenetic changes, or create helpful change. You have more control over your child's environment than you may realize. You can raise the water level by minimizing the harmful things to which your child is exposed (reducing their total load) and maximizing the ones that shore up health (increasing their total supports).

Most of the things over which you can exert some real influence fall under the headers of *food, toxins, bugs, and stress.* All of these things talk to your genes, impact your epigenetics, and shape your metabolism. Depending on your choices and your luck, they can help keep your child's lake full, or drain it out.

RESEARCH SPOTLIGHT: ALLOSTATIC LOAD AND TOTAL LOAD

Researchers use the term *allostatic load* to talk about the impact on your body of the buildup of stress from many sources. Psychologists focus on social and emotional stressors while toxicologists focus on toxic stressors. Repeated and chronic stress from different sources adds up and takes a growing toll on your cells and organs.

Stress can come from nutritional, toxic, infectious, and emotional sources. While stressors each have specific effects, they also have general effects. In some ways your body doesn't care where the stress comes from.

The cascade of difficulties Caleb experienced as an infant was a buildup of allostatic load. I use the term *total load* because all these stressors add up to make your cells, organs, and brain have a harder time and to make you more vulnerable.

Food–for Good or Bad

The classic American diet—loaded with fat, sugar, and empty calories—is a disaster for everyone, but even more so for kids with autism. Take, for example, the Pop-Tart. Nearly two billion of them are eaten annually, according to the Kellogg Company, which makes them. A single strawberry Pop-Tart contains 254 calories, its box says, but a negligible amount of iron and calcium, and absolutely no vitamin A, C, or other nutrients, according to its label. It has 1 gram of fiber out of the 25 you're supposed to consume in a day, and fewer than 3 grams of protein per serving. Eating anything with calories offers a burst of energy, but if the food lacks substantial amounts of fiber and protein, that burst is quickly followed by a crash. Routinely eating such calorie-dense, nutrient-poor foods can lead to obesity, diabetes, and even cancer. And as I will show you in the chapters ahead, these foods can make autism a lot harder to live with.

Diet and Metabolic Vulnerability

Why do we need vitamins and minerals and all-around good nutrition? Because they are the ingredients we need for our metabolism, for getting our body's work done. When we have lots of nutrients available, we have more resources for handling whatever challenges come along.

But if we're having a hard time, we'll have an even harder time with poor nutrition. It's a good guess that your child is having a difficult time getting through the day (and often also the night). You may be able to see this at the level of having problems with learning things. But think of your child's chemistry and cells. They are probably having a hard time, too. In particular your child may be in that gray area of vulnerability where your choices can influence whether they do better or worse.

Children with autism are at particular risk because of their finicky diets. The all-beige diet that many prefer (the bread, cheese, macaroni type of diet) lacks a diverse set of nutrients. They get a lot of sugar and refined flour, but not enough fiber, omega-3 fatty acids, or other essential nutrients. An "average" diet may be good enough for a healthy child but it may not be for an already challenged child on the autism spectrum. A child with autism is likely stressed much or all of the time, and stress increases nutritional needs. Digestive problems can compound these issues. So, you have to work extra hard to fortify your child.

Food Talks to Your Genes, and Genes Talk Back

Until the last century, people thought the main purpose of vitamins was to avoid deficiency diseases, such as rickets, caused by a lack of vitamin D, and scurvy, triggered by a need for C. Today many people think they're eating a nutritious diet if they meet the minimum standards set by the government's Recommended Daily Allowance, now called the Dietary Reference Intake. But these federal standards are floors—the least amount nearly everyone needs to avoid rickets and scurvy. They are not aimed at dealing with differences among individuals, because of genes or age (we have different vitamin needs at age two than at eighty-two). They also don't address differences within your own body, depending on how much sleep you get, whether you are sick, and how much stress you're under.

A new science of "nutrigenomics" has emerged to grapple with this gigantic new vision of food-gene relationships. Food can make the genome cry, or sing. It's going to be a while before we can use nutrigenomics to prescribe precise individualized diet regimens for individuals. But it's clear that we all need as rich a supply of food information as possible. It gives our bodies a large menu of choices for meeting the constantly changing demands we place on them.

Start by Reading Labels but Don't Stop There

Labels on the side of food packages can help you count the big things like calories, carbs, fats, and fiber, but they don't scratch the surface of what we now know are important nutrients. There are many vitamins and minerals not included, and there is a world of "phytonutrients" that get no mention at all. Phytonutrients are all the thousands of different chemicals in fruits and vegetables that give them their colors, flavors, and health-giving properties. These chemicals include flavonoids (found in colored fruits and vegetables, as well as dark chocolate, teas, and coffee), resveratrol (found in grapes), carotenoids (found in carrots), and lycopenes (found in tomatoes). These substances can give a boost to many of the body's chemical and immune processes that are often compromised in autism.

High Nutrient Density vs. Junk Food

The best way to give your child enough nutrients is to provide him or her with a healthy diet. More and more scientists are calling for a move to "high nutrient density" as the best approach for making decisions about what to eat. This means getting as many nutrients as possible for every calorie you consume. This is especially important for your child.

Plant-based foods—vegetables and fruits in particular—are the best sources of high nutrient density.

Packaged, processed foods are for the most part not as full of nutrients as fresh foods. They give lots of energy (calories) but not a lot of nutrients. Much of the good stuff gets sacrificed to give the product a long shelf life. Processed food is supposed to save you time. But the minutes you save may turn into hours, days, and more spent dealing with health and behavior problems. Cleaning up your diet can be hard, but it's even harder to live with a person whose diet is messing them up.

Let me quote Walter Willett, Harvard professor of nutrition and public health and author of *Eat, Drink, and Be Healthy*. He talks about adult diseases, but as I will show you, a lot of the risks for these chronic adult diseases are a problem in autism, too.

A diet rich in fruits and vegetables can: decrease the chances of having a heart attack or stroke, protect against a variety of cancers, lower blood pressure, help you avoid the painful intestinal ailment called diverticulitis, guard against two common aging-related eye diseases . . . add variety to diet and enliven your palate. . . . Pills that contain one or two or ten substances made by plants just won't do. Why not? Plants make or sequester a seemingly endless cornucopia of compounds that have biological activity in the human body. The vast majority of these phytochemicals have yet to be discovered, named, chemically characterized and biologically evaluated. . . . The odds are high that the benefits previously listed emanate from many different substances found in plants and quite possibly from the interaction of these substances.

Food: How to Get Started

In each of the next few chapters I will add and elaborate on food and nutrition information I have started laying out here. Begin now by building some awareness of your child's current reality, and what you need to think about changing.

1. Look through your cupboards and refrigerator and make an estimation of:
    a. How much of your food is packaged;
    b. How much of your food is fresh;
    c. How many fruits and vegetables you have in your house.

2. Write down what your child likes to eat and what your child refuses to eat. Take a look at the resource list at the end of this book to help you find ways to help a child who is a very picky eater. Chapter 7 will give you behavioral techniques you can use.

3. Start a food diary, or add foods to your daily log. Write down what your child eats, how your child functions (learning, behavior, focus, health) during the day and night, and how your child sleeps. In subsequent chapters I will give you more things to attend to in your diary.

4. Start learning about how to feed your child and your family whole, unprocessed foods. Fruits and vegetables are rich in vitamins, minerals, and phytonutrients, and it's particularly good to eat a "rainbow" diet, with lots of foods of different natural colors, like sweet potatoes, carrots, green vegetables, peppers, and berries.

5. Avoid the high-calorie, low-nutrient junk food usually found on the middle aisles of the grocery store. This means avoiding foods high in sugar, refined flour, trans fats, and food coloring, as well as processed (or deli) meats. Also avoid junk food that may be packaged as "natural" or "alternative."

6. Help your child gently toward eating a high-nutrient-density diet. You can start very gently. You may have to deal with your child's intolerance of strange textures and tastes. In each chapter ahead I will give more food tips, related to gut, allergy, sensory, brain, and behavior issues.

7. Buy a Vitamix or other strong, high-speed blender. Learn to make smoothies and purees. These have lots of nutrients and also lots of fiber, which is good for your child's digestion.

8. Start very gradually introducing child-friendly recipes, even as little as one teaspoonful at one time, or even less. Your child may need to see a new food at least a dozen times before they'll try more than a bite. It's okay to let them play with the food, at least sometimes—that's one of the ways they can get familiar with it.

9. Many parents find that a zinc supplement increases their child's interest in new foods. Zinc can enhance taste sensitivity.

10. To hedge against vitamin shortfalls, particularly with a finicky eater, it's a good idea to provide a daily multivitamin and

multimineral supplement and to address any levels that are unusually low.

SMOOTHIES, PUREES, AND BROTHS

You can make high-nutrient-density purees of vegetables, beans, or fruits and give them to your child or mix them in with your child's other foods, starting with a small amount at a time, even as little as a quarter teaspoonful. Then build up gradually.

A Vitamix or similar high-speed blender lets you turn raw vegetables as hard as carrots, celery, and broccoli into drinks or purees just by adding water or other liquid.

Blended and pureed foods are easier to digest, because the nutrients are more accessible. Smoothies can also be fast and easy to make.

Smoothies

Fruit smoothies can be very tasty. Some vegetable combinations can be tasty, too. Start with raw or frozen ingredients if you can.

Green Smoothies

Green smoothies are especially loaded with vitamins, minerals, and phytonutrients that can greatly build your child's health and resilience. You can mix and match raw green leafy vegetables with fruits and water or other liquids. Some examples are spinach and pears, kale and mango, swiss chard, cilantro, and blueberries. You can find many more recipes on the Web—or use your imagination!

Purees

Vegetable purees, bean purees, sauces, spreads, and dips can be made with a variety of ingredients and used in many ways.

Broths

Vegetable broths can be made by boiling vegetables for several hours and then straining out the solids. Bone broths, a staple in many traditional cultures as well as in high-class French cuisine, involve simmering bones with vegetables for up to twenty-four hours and then straining. You can use these broths as bases for your blended and pureed foods to further increase their nutrient density. Make extra and store in your freezer in containers, or in ice cube trays so you can pop them into dishes you're cooking. The cookbook *Nourishing Traditions* has further instructions for making broths.

Toxins

No one is free of toxins. I am using the word *toxins* here broadly, to include not only natural and chemical substances but also other man-made exposures, such as radiation, that can have a harmful physical impact on your genes and metabolism. Not all chemicals or exposures are necessarily harmful. But given the amount of chemicals and other things human beings have invented at an accelerating rate over the past two centuries, it is surprising how many holes there are in our knowledge about the health impacts of these creations.

Even though there are upwards of eighty-five thousand chemicals being produced, we have little data about their impact on our health and even less on children's health, according to a 2006 study published in *The Lancet.* Currently there is no requirement to screen chemicals for their impact on the developing brain; as a result only twenty to thirty chemicals have undergone such testing before hitting store shelves. In essence, we are flying blind about what risks these substances are posing to our babies and children. And yet the whole scientific field of developmental neurotoxicology supports the idea that the developing brain is exquisitely vulnerable to toxic impacts.

Among the things you should know but may not:

1. There may be no lowest level of impact below which a chemical can be considered "safe" for everyone. Exposures may have an impact on our genetic and cellular molecules at extremely low levels, even one ten-thousandth or more lower than what might previously have been considered the toxic threshold.
2. Toxins at even low levels can change which genes turn on and off.

3. Toxins can damage genes.

4. Toxins can look similar to your body's own chemical signal molecules and can confuse your body about which one said what.

5. Toxic exposures at very low levels can change the way the brain develops from earliest fetal life through toddlerhood, and even beyond.

6. Toxins do things in combination that can't be predicted by what they do by themselves. But testing is one chemical at a time; almost none of our safety testing looks at combinations of substances.

7. The cord blood of babies contains at least trace amounts of hundreds of chemicals, meaning babies have already been exposed while in the womb. There is plenty of science showing that even low levels of exposure during this time creates vulnerability to epigenetic changes—that is, altered gene expression. We know almost nothing about the long-term impacts.

Toxins Add Drag Every Day

Toxins don't impact only early development. They can affect function every day by actively interfering with metabolism. They can slow down or block enzymes, making cells sluggish. They can interfere with the absorption of nutrients, creating insufficient supplies. They can interfere with many different kinds of cellular activities. Poorer function can be stressful, and stress ramps up nutritional needs even further. This is a vicious circle that entraps many children with autism as well as many other people who are chronically ill.

Toxins can also send confusing molecular signals. Certain chemicals that have the same shape as our own natural hormones, called endocrine disrupters, confuse the body into thinking the brain sent it a hormonal signal. Some common chemicals that are endocrine disrupters include DDT, PCBs, PBDEs from flame retardants (which can be sprayed on everything from kids' pajamas to living room sofas), bisphenol A in some plastic bottles, and phthalates, which are in a variety of household products. Researchers are studying whether endocrine disruption could be a factor in autism's apparent gender bias with diagnoses going to four boys for every one girl.

CHILDREN ARE AT HIGHER RISK FOR EXPOSURE

Children are generally exposed to more toxins than adults. Children spend more time on the floor than adults, kicking up, breathing, and swallowing the dust and dirt that collects there. They put all kinds of things in their mouths that adults are never exposed to. They get sick from germs to which adults are already immune. They take more medications to get rid of those, including antibiotics that kill off helpful microbes along with the bad. And, of course, all these exposures happen simultaneously. Their bodies are smaller, their detox systems aren't fully mature, and they have more skin surface per pound than adults do—making them more vulnerable to exposures that come in through the skin.

All of this applies even more to children who may have extra vulnerabilities from their genes, or from not feeling well, such as children with autism. It may take fewer exposures for a child with autism to have problems than a child with no autism. When a toxin or bug targets an area of genetic weakness, that gene-environment interaction can make a much bigger impact.

Toxin Inventory: Aim for Prudence and Precaution

What should you do in the face of this risk we don't fully understand? You might want to learn about the *precautionary principle*. This is the idea that public policy about exposures should demand proof of safety ahead of time, rather than waiting until harm becomes apparent. Harm takes a long time to prove—look at how long it took to regulate cigarettes or to take lead out of gasoline.

You can also take a prudent, precautionary approach in your life. I think a precautionary approach is the right way to go for your child (and for you and your whole family). Go for the lowest amount of expo-

THE PRECAUTIONARY PRINCIPLE

The Precautionary Principle was defined in the Wingspread Statement, produced in 1998 at a landmark three-day academic conference of scientists, scholars, and activists convened by the Science and Environmental Health Network. Europeans use this principle as the basis for their chemical policy.

"When an activity raises threats of harm to human health or the environment, precautionary measures should be taken even if some cause and effect relationships are not fully established scientifically."

sures you can manage without making yourself crazy. Here are some suggestions for doing this:

1. Take a walk around your house and look at all the places where you are using chemical-based substances. Likely places to look are under your sinks, in your toiletries, in your cosmetics, in your garage or utility closet, and in your laundry area. I am increasingly convinced that it's worth the extra few dollars to buy products made from botanicals, or to make household products yourself out of natural substances like baking soda and lemon. (For guides to less hazardous products, go to the Environmental Working Group's website, ewg.org. For cleaning product recipes, I like EarthEasy.com.)

2. Think about other sources of exposures in your child's life, like school and play areas. One way to minimize dust or other contaminants you may bring into the house: Leave shoes at the door.

3. Some states and school districts are forbidding the use of pesticides in schools and school yards. Find out about the policies in your community.

4. Learn about the water quality in your community, or in your well. Find out whether there is lead in your pipes. Consider using a quality water filter. There are filters for your sink, your showerhead, and your whole house.

5. Avoid toxins in your food. These can include preservatives, additives, pesticides, and more.
6. Learn about sources of toxic exposure in your community.
7. If you are thinking about detoxifying your child, hold on. In the next chapter, I will tell you more about how our own bodies can detox naturally, how those processes can get stuck, and what you can do about it.

Bugs

Infectious agents—bacteria, viruses, fungus, parasites (or "bugs," for short)—are a part of our environment. Some of them can make us sick, and some of them are vital to our health. Like us, these bugs are also influenced by their environment. When bacteria and viruses face challenges like chemical or antibiotic stress, one of their responses is to swap genes with one another, mixing and matching to become "fit" enough to survive. We see this as antibiotic or antiparasitic resistance, in which the bugs can become resistant to treatment, making drugs ineffective.

Your child's vulnerability to bugs is a function not only of how infectious the bug is, but also of how strong or weak his or her own system is. That's another reason to keep your child's system as robust as possible with healthy foods and minimal toxic exposures.

To help, you can make a list of your child's infections, tracking:
a. How many infections your child has had and how many have been treated by antibiotics or other drugs;
b. How infections have affected your child's diet, sleep, and behavior;
c. Whether anything else happened before, during, or after the infection that you see in a new light after having read this chapter and the last one.

Stress Isn't Just for Grown-ups

Stress happens when there's more going on than you have the resources to handle. Stress is not just about emotional overload; it's about biological overload, too. Stress can be caused by lack of adequate sleep, anxiety, illness, and toxins—or a combination of all four. Just as someone who gets laid off will have more stress if they have no family or community support, toxins and illnesses cause your body more stress if you've been eating or sleeping poorly, or are prone to worrying. Those anxious tendencies, which could be influenced by genes as well as by shallow breathing, too much caffeine, a bad diet, and an inability to relax, will make some people more vulnerable to stresses than others.

Think of your autistic child and how many sources of stress he or she has: If he has communication issues, he will not be able to communicate his needs, which adds stress. If she isn't sleeping well, exhaustion will aggravate her immune problems. If he's a picky eater, he won't get enough nutrients and gut problems mean he may not even be absorbing what little he does eat. All these things add to your child's stress burden—their total load—and their need for support at every level.

Over the next several chapters, I will walk you through how all these problems—triggered by biological and environmental stresses—can pile up and in turn cause more biological and brain stress. But for now, I want you to understand how poor food and toxins can make these problems worse, and how good food and safe products can make them better.

KEEP IN MIND

- Genes create risk for autism and sometimes it's high risk.
- Environment creates risk for autism and sometimes it's high risk.
- Genes and environment may also lower risk for autism.
- "Environment" includes all experiences with food, toxins, bugs, and stress—all the things that happen to us in daily life.
- Our daily choices may shape our gene expression.
- Our daily choices may cause or prevent gene damage.
- The total load of genetic vulnerabilities plus harmful environmental exposures is probably what turns risk into autism.
- When the environment promotes health, it takes more risk and total load to get in trouble.
- When the environment creates risk, it takes less total load or genetic vulnerability to get in trouble.

But also remember

- No single environmental factor causes autism.
- No specific toxin or any specific intervention, such as vaccinations, has been shown to cause autism.
- Genes are not more important than environment; nor is environment more important than genes.

PART II

Protect and Nourish the Whole Body: From Vicious Circles to Resilience

CHAPTER 3

Repair and Support Cells and Cycles

To get better, Ana Todd first had to get worse. Much worse. When she was twenty-six, Ana was diagnosed with chronic fatigue syndrome, on top of her autism. She couldn't get out of bed, had to take a leave of absence from work, and didn't know how she would survive. She felt so lousy, she says, that she was willing to do pretty much anything to get better.

Ana had been diagnosed with autism at age three, because of her repetitive behaviors, language difficulties, and an awkwardness that made other children think she was strange. She knew from a very early age that they were right.

Throughout her childhood, Ana had been physically awkward, always the last picked for teams in school, always bumping into things. Diarrhea, stomach pains, and illness plagued her. She had whooping cough when she was no more than four months old, and seemed sick from that point onward. She had scarlet fever and middle ear infections before her autism diagnosis; more infections and chicken pox before she turned nine. Then, most of her physical problems seemed to clear up until her early twenties.

As a child, she was a strong reader and writer but had a terrible time keeping up with conversations—she wanted to interact with others, but it was always an exhausting struggle. "Talking to other people was a bit like being on a phone line that was always cutting out," she says. "You'd put together the story the best that you could and hope that it made sense, and hope that you hadn't missed things, or misinterpreted things. Obviously, that was extremely distressing and caused me a lot of anxiety."

Speaking was equally stressful. Ana would have a clear idea of what she wanted to say, but when she opened her mouth the words would come out jumbled. A simple sentence like "How are you today?" might instead start "Today are . . ." And then she would realize she had stumbled, and would get tongue-tied trying to get it right, muttering "um," "arrh," or "nn" as she struggled.

Ana became terribly anxious and socially withdrawn. As a teenager, she was so depressed she spent some time in a mental institution. It was there that she realized no one else could help her get better—she had to figure it out for herself.

That sense of self-reliance was still with her a decade later when she began to spiral downward, with less and less strength for everyday activities. Again she was sick seemingly all the time. After about nine months of dragging herself to doctor after doctor, Ana was diagnosed with chronic fatigue syndrome. Something had pushed her body over the edge from troubled to truly disabled.

In this chapter I want to propose that whatever the push was, it built on vulnerabilities at every level of Ana's body. As a small child, Ana had been diagnosed with autism, but her childhood had been peppered with medical illnesses, too. Her whole-body problems from childhood resurfaced in her young adult chronic fatigue.

It took her a year to find a doctor who could do more than tell her it was "all in her head." That doctor believed her problems started in her cells—all over her body. When Ana's chronic fatigue syndrome was treated at the cellular level, her autism melted away. And she transformed herself from an awkward, obsessive, clumsy, anxious person into a self-possessed woman who is happy with her life and looking forward to the future.

Ana did not simply have a mind problem causing her fatigue, or a brain problem causing her autism. She had a whole-body health problem causing both. Autism is a condition of the whole body, including the brain, starting at its smallest unit, the cell. Cells are the basis of everything our mind, brain, and bodies do. I want to take you on a tour of the body's cells to see what might have gone wrong inside Ana's, what might be going wrong in your child's, and what Ana has done to make her cells—and her life—work better.

Getting into Cells

Having a child with autism gives you a pressing need to know about cells and how they work. You might have first learned about cells and chemistry in high school biology class. Back then these terms were probably just words you had to memorize and cartoon-like pictures of circles with things inside them. Now cells may hold a key to improving your child's health. So let's try to make friends with these cells and get inside their world.

Cells are like houses. They are safe spaces shielded from the outside by a membrane, like the walls of the house. They have information detectors in their cells, like windows that keep an eye on what's happening outside, and an elaborate internal signal system to alert everyone inside to get ready for guests or intruders. Different signals are sent if there's a need for food or if viruses (burglars) are in the house making trouble. Inside the cell lots of things get done to keep the cell alive; these things happen in different membrane-enclosed areas, like rooms. Cells even have trash disposals, and little furnaces (called mitochondria) to keep them warm and make energy. The health of your child's cells depends on all these parts (and more) being able to stay connected to one another and do their jobs well.

The cells' health can be compromised by genetic mutations. They can also be threatened by two basic supply problems: *not enough* and *too much.*

Not enough: If the cells don't get enough food and nutrients to make energy they will get sluggish. If they don't get enough nutrients to drive enzymes they will get inefficient at things like taking out the trash, sending signals, and using food. If they don't get enough of the right kinds of supplies their pipes will spring leaks, potholes will open up in the driveway, and walls will begin to crumble.

Too much: If the cells get too much food, their switches and signals for figuring out what they need will get confused. If the ingredients are of poor quality, things won't work right and will wear out too soon. If the cells get too many toxins or are overloaded with stress, their trash removal equipment will get stuck, and nasty crud will pile up, making the cells less healthy.

In this chapter I'm going to focus on two key functions of the cells: making energy and taking out the trash. These processes are vulnerable in everyone. There's genetic evidence that some or many people with autism may have even greater vulnerability here. And research suggests there are also simple and practical things you can do to reduce the severity of these problems.

Troublemakers in the Power Plant

Every cell has mitochondria, though cells whose work demands high energy have more mitochondria than cells with quieter jobs. These tiny furnaces take sugars and transform them step by step into little packages of energy that fuel all the cell's other activities. Problems with the mitochondria create problems for the whole cell and the whole body—in particular for the brain, which uses huge amounts of energy.

What can go wrong in our precious mitochondrial power plants?

HOW MITOCHONDRIA WORK

Mitochondria create heat, but they can't stand to get too hot themselves. To keep the heat under control, they make fuel out of high-energy sugar molecules in tiny, well-controlled steps, each of which extracts just a little bit of energy. The energy is then stored in molecules called ATP that can be used around the cell to get things done. There are three basic parts of the cell's energy-generating machinery:

The first, most ancient part of the machinery doesn't require oxygen—it's "anaerobic." When you get sore after exercise, some of the soreness comes from the lactic acid that is the end product of this first phase. In fact, being "out of shape" means among other things that your energy machinery is weak; and "getting fit" involves building up your mitochondria so they can keep up with more and more exercise.

The next step of energy generation is the citric acid cycle, also called the Krebs cycle after the scientist who discovered it. This is the circular, eight-step pathway you probably learned about in high school biology. Each step coaxes a little more energy out of the molecules and stores it in carrier molecules called NAD and FAD.

The last step is called the electron transport chain. In this process, the carrier molecules pass through five energy-releasing states, capturing the energy released in each.

Like the triggers we discussed earlier, food, toxins, bugs, and stress are again the culprits. And as before, genes play a role as well.

Genes: Every step in the energy production process is made possible by enzymes—proteins made up of amino acids. The order of the amino acids is determined by DNA. A mutation in the DNA may change the order of the amino acids, and the chemical properties of the enzyme may change, too. A dramatic shift in the order can lead to "mitochondrial disease," which is a serious and sometimes fatal problem. Other mutations can slow things down or speed things up in more subtle ways that aren't even noticeable until more demand is put on the system.

Food: Your mitochondria need you to eat a healthy, balanced diet so they'll have the supplies they need to make energy out of enzymes. Many enzymes in the energy production process require vitamin and mineral helpers. Some big players are the B vitamins (NAD and FAD are made using B vitamins), magnesium, and zinc. Shortages of these ingredients can occur when supply doesn't keep up with demand.

Toxins: Thousands of toxins, including chemicals and heavy metals, can interfere with various steps along the way. Steps in the energy production Krebs cycle can be slowed down by toxins, and the electron transport chain can be stopped dead by toxins at many places. Thousands of medications can also slow down the mitochondria's energy-producing process. Some of the side effects of drugs come from their impacts on mitochondria.

Bugs: Bacteria and viruses can increase demand on mitochondria because fighting infections takes energy. Bugs can also compete with our own cells for energy, or interfere with the mitochondria directly. Some bugs produce toxins that disrupt our biochemistry, including energy production. And some of the antibiotics we use to fight infections target the bacteria's energy systems, to weaken or kill the invaders. This can sometimes spill over and injure our own energy machinery.

Stress: Being stressed, whether we missed the train, have too much to do, or are fighting a cold, takes energy. Such a strain on the system occurs at every level of the body, from molecules, cells, organs, and brain to your whole system. When your cells experience more demand than they can handle, they need to shift into a defensive or protective mode, and this diverts resources from normal, everyday activities. Over time this wears down the health of your cells. Your mitochondria may not be able to keep up with this demand.

Mitochondrial Problems in Autism

Research clearly connecting mitochondrial disease or dysfunction to autism is still in its early stages. We do know that at least a subset of people with autism have mitochondrial problems. While some of these problems may be caused by genes ("primary" mitochondrial disease), much may be caused by environment ("secondary" mitochondrial dysfunction), according to research published in the prestigious *Journal of the American Medical Association* in 2010. Other studies have shown that mitochondria are very vulnerable to environmental injury. Environmental influences might drag your mitochondria down into a "gray zone"—not diseased, but not healthy, either—without outright poisoning or killing you. So might mild genetic mutations.

RESEARCH SPOTLIGHT: MITOCHONDRIA AND AUTISM

According to mitochondrial specialist John Jay Gargus, many studies have shown that a large number of people with autism have "gray zone" problems with mitochondria—mild but still troublesome.

Researchers Daniel Rossignol and Richard Frye recently looked systematically at 112 studies that explored a possible link between autism and mitochondrial disease. They found that about 1 out of every 20 people with autism had mitochondrial disease, compared to 1 of 10,000 people in the general population.

Many more, as many as 1 in 3 of those with autism, showed some biological evidence of mitochondrial dysfunction that did not rise to the level of "disease." And nearly 80 percent of those who had diagnosable mitochondrial disease didn't show any indications of genetic abnormalities.

Although many more studies need to be done to flesh this out, the research suggests that mitochondrial problems are far more common in autism than in the general population, and that they don't need to reach levels of serious disease to have an impact. The lack of clear genetic cause in most cases suggests they may be triggered by a person's environment.

Could Ana Todd's clumsiness, lack of energy, and communication difficulties be related to mitochondrial problems? We can't prove this in her particular case, but we can wonder, since she responded so well to treatments that could have energized her struggling mitochondria.

Sweeping Up the Dirt

When cells "invented" the Krebs cycle about 3.5 billion years ago, the extra energy enabled them to thrive and grow bigger. The Krebs cycle allowed an explosion of new life-forms. But it came with a trade-off. The oxygen that fueled the cycle was unstable. By-products of these unstable molecules, known as "free radicals," wandered around the cell sticking to things and causing damage. Cells evolved a way to keep the dangerous oxygen under control—so-called antioxidants, which sop up the free radicals.

Antioxidants work like flypaper, with free radicals sticking to them and then getting tossed out of the body with them. If you're short on major antioxidants like vitamin C, E, or glutathione, you won't clear out as many free radicals. Bad habits and bad environment—poor diet, smoking, pollution, toxins, drugs, stress, radiation, trauma, aging, and infections—can all deplete your antioxidants. And shortages of vitamins B_6, B_{12}, or folate, zinc, or magnesium can keep your body from being able to make its own antioxidants like glutathione, the most powerful of the body's antioxidants. Antioxidants like vitamin C are found freely in colorful fruits and vegetables, but most Americans don't eat enough of these healthy foods to keep up with the free radicals our bodies produce.

When free radicals aren't removed, you get into a situation called "oxidative stress," which can cause damage to DNA and cells. In 2008, researchers at the Massachusetts General Hospital surveyed recent studies on oxidative stress and showed a link between this stress and a variety of psychiatric conditions. Oxidative stress is also present in many chronic and degenerative diseases including asthma, diabetes, cancer, obesity, Alzheimer's, and Parkinson's. It is not surprising, then, to learn that oxidative stress is present in autism as well.

Abha and Ved Chauhan and W. Ted Brown of the New York State Institute for Basic Research in Developmental Disabilities have launched a large research program studying oxidative stress in autism. So far they

FOOD SOURCES OF ANTIOXIDANTS

- Berries, including blueberries, blackberries, raspberries, strawberries, and cranberries
- Beans, such as kidney, pinto, and black beans
- Fruits, including many apple varieties (with peel), avocados, cherries, green and red pears, fresh or dried plums, pineapple, kiwi, and others
- Vegetables, such as artichokes, spinach, red cabbage, red and white potatoes (with peel), sweet potatoes, and broccoli
- Beverages, including green tea, coffee, red wine, and fruit juices that are rich in color
- Nuts, such as walnuts, pistachios, pecans, hazelnuts, and almonds
- Herbs, including ground cloves, cinnamon, ginger, dried oregano leaf, and turmeric powder
- Dark chocolate

Source: Mayo Clinic

and others have found oxidative stress present in many children with autism, as well as in brain tissue of people with autism. Their research shows that people who lost language were most likely to show evidence of oxidative stress.

Oxidative stress can also cause mitochondrial damage. Several studies have found markers of oxidative stress damage to the mitochondria's vulnerable cell membranes in urine samples from people with autism. Here's another of our vicious circles: The more the mitochondrial membranes are injured, the less able the mitochondria are to repair the damage.

Taking Out the Trash

Cells need to take out the garbage, including toxins. Cells make toxin by-products as part of their work. They also have to deal with toxins that get dumped on them from the body's environmental exposures. But, just as it takes some effort to put your trash in bags and bring it to the curb, so it takes some work for cells. This dirty work is often done by sulfur, which is "sticky" enough to grab on to waste and heavy metals and flush them out of the body.

Two amino acids that contain sulfur—cysteine and methionine—are also important in making the antioxidant and detox molecule glutathione. If glutathione gets used up, or if your body has problems making it, a lot of jobs don't get done right.

Your liver, which is the body's major trash disposal unit, makes a lot of glutathione. It also has lots of other chemicals to turn toxins into

RESEARCH SPOTLIGHT: METHYLATION

S. Jill James at the University of Arkansas found that if you have several gene mutations in the production line (or pathway) that makes glutathione, you are at higher risk for autism. This pathway also supports methylation, which is important to many things, including making neurotransmitters, helping build cell membranes, and controlling gene expression.

The methylation pathway helps the body handle toxins and immune problems. But toxins can slow down or block this pathway. This is a vicious circle.

This pathway starts with the amino acid methionine, which is important to obtain from food to keep methylation moving. Several nutrients such as methylcobalamin (a form of vitamin B_{12}), vitamin B_6, and folinic acid (a B vitamin) are important to this pathway and may help unblock a stuck system. Research in autism and other conditions gives some support to the idea that supplementation with these nutrients may reduce methylation pathway problems. More studies are under way. Research also shows that low methylation, which increases risk for cancer and other diseases, can be avoided by a diet high in vegetables and fruits.

forms that are easily removed from the cell or the body. Think about a dirty dish covered with oil. You can't get it clean if you just rinse it with water. But if you add soap, the soap changes the oil into a form that can be washed off. The liver puts many of these repackaged toxins into bile, which is then passed out of your body in stool (which happens to be what largely accounts for stool's color).

Caught in Vicious Circles

Genetic glitches, oxidative stress, mitochondrial dysfunction, weakened repair systems all feed on one another and make problems worse. Oxidative stress, for instance, interferes with production of a key enzyme, methionine synthase, that helps produce glutathione. But since glutathione is essential for cell repair, trash removal, and recovery from oxidative stress, once damage starts, it becomes a vicious circle that can feed on itself.

Ana Todd's symptoms indicate that her body was overrun by these vicious circles. Remember her weakened immune system, both in early childhood and again just before she came down with chronic fatigue syndrome? Oxidative stress can sap the immune system. And a tired immune system is a setup for more oxidative stress.

Ana also walked with heavy, dragging footsteps—her husband used to tease her about how loud they were. She says she walked this way because it took so much effort to lift her feet off the floor. Having such heavy footsteps can be a sign of low energy, which could be a symptom of mitochondrial dysfunction, as could be the fatigue that tied her to her bed. If you've ever had a day when you were too tired to lift your feet up off the floor, you'll remember how much that dragged you down emotionally, too.

Toxins almost definitely made things worse for Ana. She grew up in an industrial town, and her childhood home backed up onto a regional airport. The air often smelled like a steel mill, she says. Tests in her mid-twenties revealed that Ana's bloodstream had high levels of contaminants from jet fuel and heavy metals found only in industry.

Her diet probably contributed, too. She had always been an extremely picky eater. Milk, potatoes, and pasta were her dietary staples. She had stomach pain for most of her life, which only went away when she switched to a gluten-free diet. She says she first heard about gluten-free diets for autism when she was about nineteen—and she thought it sounded ridiculous. "I remember talking to my mother, saying: 'How can a condition as complex as autism possibly be solved by diet?'" Now, she says she doesn't like the hyper, physically awkward person she becomes when she eats gluten. It's really not worth it, she says. Recently, she tried avoiding sugar as well. "I felt amazing. I didn't feel hyperactive or silly."

Ana's story, like those of many people with autism, also suggests that her body could cope better at some times than at others. She had her good days, where she could talk fluently, only stumbling a few times, "whereas a bad day was when I would jumble up every single sentence."

Treating Health Rather than Disease

Seeing someone as seriously ill as Ana get better calls for an examination of what she did. It doesn't seem like much in comparison to how sick she was—but little things can accomplish a lot.

After spending a year looking for a doctor who could help, Ana finally found Dr. Robyn Cosford, an integrative physician who blends conventional medicine and complementary methods. Cosford's approach was basically the same as I am suggesting: to avoid or minimize new toxic, infectious, and allergic exposures; and to strengthen Ana's body's own ability to renew itself and rid itself of oxidative stress and toxins. In other words, the goal was not so much to treat disease, but more to promote health.

To accomplish that, Dr. Cosford had Ana:

- Take a specially formulated multivitamin
- Take additional supplements including cod liver oil, folinic acid, and Saint-John's-wort
- Drink a juice extremely high in antioxidants and phytonutrients every morning and evening
- Use products to help her handle exposure to electromagnetic frequencies that seem to bother her
- Eat a diet free of gluten and casein
- Take homeopathic remedies.

I will explain the rationale behind each of these recommendations shortly, but first let me tell you what happened when Ana started following this regimen.

A Transformation

Ana says her chronic fatigue symptoms faded first. Then, as she regained her energy, she realized that her treatment was impacting her autism, too. Ana is certain that if she were tested for autism today, she wouldn't fit the diagnosis. It's been about three years since she first started making changes in her diet, and at age twenty-nine, she says her body is still changing for the better.

During her mid-twenties, Ana says, she was able to mask many of her autistic symptoms, and worked in a place she described as a magnet for nerdy people and probably others on the spectrum. In that context, her behaviors didn't seem so abnormal, she says. She met and married her husband while working there.

One day early in her recovery from chronic fatigue, Ana noticed that she was walking into walls, spilling things on herself, and—weirdest of all—reaching for something and missing it by a few inches. This lasted about two weeks. Then it went away, leaving her more coordinated than she'd ever been.

Ana thinks the temporary awkwardness was her body getting used to a new level of coordination. While her body was recomputing its routines, it was pretty confused. Now that it's corrected itself, she's a better driver, she says (though still not the best, she admits, laughing), with improved coordination and faster reflexes. Her heavy, scraping footsteps are gone now, too.

It was a few months into her treatment when Ana realized her speech wasn't as tortured as it had been before. Her awkward speech "just sort of seemed to melt away without me even recognizing it." Now, she says, she doesn't trip over words any more than others do. (In a two-hour conversation with me, the only word she stumbled on was *dyspraxia*, the medical term for the awkward speech patterns that plagued her—an irony that left her giggling with amusement.)

Clearer speech has also improved her anxiety and obsessiveness. Now, no longer worrying about whether she is going to say something awkward or stupid, she can relax about other things. As she puts it: "My anxiety is melting away to nothing . . . I can let things go. I don't go over things over and over again in my brain." She used to stress out, for instance, if the clothespins she used for hanging her wash on the line didn't match. Now she doesn't care.

She also noticed some less welcome changes—the loss of certain skills and talents, which returned as she continued to improve. Ana had always prided herself on her writing ability, but about eighteen months into her treatment she found she was unable to write clearly anymore. Her writing resembled her speech at its most convoluted. "I was like 'Oh my God, what is happening, what happens if I never get it back?'" A year and a half later, her writing skills are better than they were before, but for a few months while her immune system acted up, her quantitative skills slipped, too. A two-week vacation helped her immune system bounce back, and her math skills have improved as well. She says she's perky in the morning again, and her analytical skills seem to be on the upswing.

And though her autistic memory rarely failed her—she could always impress people with her knowledge of trivia—Ana claims she's becoming more neurotypically forgetful now, as her autism symptoms fade. She's also had to redefine herself, to develop a new self-image. "All the nutty things I used to do, that's who I was. Now I'm learning it's not a loss because there's a different way of still being me."

Evaluating Treatment Options

How can Ana's experience be explained? Typically people don't get over their chronic fatigue and they certainly don't usually lose their autism symptoms in their late twenties.

I don't think anyone should use Ana's story as a recipe to follow step by step, because every person is unique. But telling you about the things she tried gives me a way to discuss the pros and cons—and evidence or lack thereof—for various approaches: the ones I think could be a good idea to try yourself, and those you may hear about on the Internet and with which I believe you should familiarize yourself.

The lesson for you is that even in circumstances where you are offered unorthodox medical treatments, it is possible to evaluate them for their advisability, in consultation with your child's doctor.

It's important to remember that the treatments Ana took were for treating her chronic fatigue, not her autism. Yet the autism went away by itself during the process. Many doctors believe, like Ana's Dr. Cosford, that autism, chronic fatigue, and a variety of other chronic illnesses all involve a deterioration of the biological systems that help us cope with the environment. To Cosford and others, the autism is not a "thing" or "specific disease" but the way the brain and body behave when their cells are having a hard time. Their treatment is therefore aimed not at the specific diseases but at the underlying biological and cellular abnormalities. That is, *these doctors aim to get the cells to work better.* Although they expect the autism or other chronic illnesses to respond, their main goal is to restore overall health.

Here is a checklist (inspired by an article in the journal *Pediatrics*) that you can use to assess treatment options you hear about:

1. Is there good biological evidence that it is effective?
   a. In autism
   b. In conditions with similar biology
   c. In animal models
   d. Biologically plausible but there's been no testing
   e. No evidence at all

2. Do we know whether it's safe?
    a. Proven safe
    b. Generally recognized as safe
    c. Risk likely to be low
    d. Possible risk or dangers
    e. Documented risk or dangers
3. How much does it cost?
    a. Free or nearly free
    b. Inexpensive
    c. Moderately expensive
    d. Extremely expensive

A proven or plausible treatment without risk and at low cost could very well be worth a try. An example of this is Epsom salt baths (the same kind of bath that athletes take when they get sore after workouts). Epsom salts, which are absorbed through the skin during a bath, are made of magnesium and sulfate, two substances very important to cell and detoxification biology. The salts' effectiveness is biologically plausible, they are generally recognized as safe, and they are very inexpensive and available over the counter in any drugstore. Many parents swear by them for helping their child calm down and sleep better, and for helping erase the dark circles under the youngster's eyes. The bath can make a very nice nighttime ritual with little if any downside.

On the other hand, a risky treatment with slim or no evidence that costs a lot of money is something you should avoid unless you can make an extremely strong and well-researched case for doing it, you fully understand the risks, and you are under the supervision of a highly experienced, serious, and competent physician—or if you are doing it as part of a reputable, institutionally approved research study. Stem cell therapy is an example of a treatment that does not make biological sense to me for autism, is wildly expensive (in part because it's not legal in the United States), has made some kids whom I know worse, and carries a high risk of danger. I would avoid it.

In between these extremes are lots of options that are harder to evaluate. Given that it may be years before even the simplest of these treatments is tested systematically, it is asking a lot that you do nothing while waiting for science to give you a hand. And it is hard to avoid hearing about tantalizing new treatments from your friends or the Internet. My advice here is to start with the simplest, cheapest, and safest approaches— and especially to build a solid foundation with high-nutrient-density, plant-based food. If you feel the need to explore riskier territory, please think hard, do lots of research, analyze critically, and monitor what you are doing extremely carefully.

Ana's Path

Let's assess Ana's treatment strategy (I'll save the diet and homeopathic remedies for the next chapter, and look at the rest here):

Multivitamin: Ana's daily vitamin included the full range of B vitamins to support mitochondrial and other basic cellular functions. It also included glutamine, glycine, and N-acetylcysteine (NAC) to support liver detoxification and glutathione production. It included several minerals: magnesium, zinc, selenium, and molybdenum, which are all exceedingly important in cellular metabolism, are often low in the general population, and are particularly important in cellular processes that may be compromised in autism. These nutrients are usually compromised in chronic illness and supplementing them can help rebuild cellular resiliency.

Many multivitamin formulations are safe and low risk, though they can be expensive and it's hard to find everything in one pill. There is always the possibility that a specific multivitamin formulation will contain too much of some nutrient for a particular person—or too little. The alternative, of putting together a cocktail of individual supplements, has the advantage of allowing you to add one at a time to assess for adverse reactions to individual components. But this can come at a much higher cost, require you to feed your child a boatload of pills, and still not really overcome the risk of an imprecise dose. Yet another alternative is to have your doctor prescribe a custom formulation made by a compounding pharmacy, but this is expensive and generally done only when a patient has unusual needs that can't be met in other ways.

Some supplements have doses many times the recommended daily allowance of certain nutrients. Some mitochondrial disease specialists prescribe cocktails of vitamins that are cofactors in the mitochondrial pathways, such as vitamins B_1 and B_2, coenzyme Q10, and carnitine.

Evidence for this practice is mixed and there is a wide variety of opinion among conventional mitochondrial disease specialists about this practice.

It's a good idea to introduce supplements one at a time and observe reactions for three to seven days before making any additional changes. That way, if there's a reaction—good or bad—you'll know where it's likely coming from. Keep a record in your log of supplements and medications, and of any reactions (see sample forms in the appendix).

Is it possible to tell precisely how much of each nutrient is needed? Generally not. We don't know enough about the nutrients. And nutritional needs may vary from day to day. So any dose is an approximation and this will remain true for the foreseeable future.

NUTRITIONAL TESTING

Can testing help you identify supplements your child might need or should avoid? The young science of nutrigenomics aims to meet this testing need in the future. For now, certain basic deficiencies can be identified, for example, of iron, but finding excesses can sometimes be tricky. Many children with autism have very low zinc levels, and if you supplement with zinc and a lab test tells you you've overshot, you should take it seriously and dial back, because too much zinc can be harmful.

Sometimes lab values may look high only because the nutrient isn't getting absorbed into the cells, and is instead piling up in the blood. It takes substantial training to tell what a high lab value really means. Even "normal" can be hard to pin down, because deficiencies or "insufficiencies" are so common in the general population, and nutritional research is tedious, expensive, and hard to fund. It's hard to tightly control these studies because nutrients come in foods and people's diets vary.

Integrative and alternative doctors may offer you complex nutritional assessment testing that goes far beyond what a pediatrician or primary care doctor following standard procedures would offer. Many mainstream doctors find these assessments disturbing or consider them to be junk science, and think they are all done in uncertified labs by unreliable methods. (Some of these independent labs are certified by the federal government through the Clinical Laboratory Improvement Amendments, for which they have to pass rigorous assessments.) If you choose to pursue these lab tests, which can cost from a few hundred to a few thousand dollars, you need to understand that they are based upon a different philosophy and set of assumptions. Their intent is less to diagnose specific diseases and more to map the "gray zone" of nutritional and metabolic vulnerability, to identify excesses and insufficiencies in relation to each person's individual needs (not necessarily deficiencies in relation to the official *Dietary Reference Intake*—what used to be known as the *Recommended Daily Allowance* or RDA).

I think that the value of these lab tests is heavily dependent upon the knowledge base of the person interpreting them. It is not always easy to find someone with strong knowledge and experience.*

* The most comprehensive source of information on these kinds of lab tests is the textbook *Laboratory Evaluations for Integrative and Functional Medicine,* second edition, published in Duluth, Georgia, by Metametrix Institute (2008) and edited by Richard Lord and J. Alexander Bralley.

Some particular nutrients in Ana's multivitamin/multimineral supplement deserve special note so you understand their purpose, since they are not in all commercial formulations.

- NAC—N-acetylcysteine is a form of the sulfur amino acid cysteine that is needed to make glutathione. In an inhaled form called Mucomyst it is currently used as a treatment for RSV, a common respiratory virus. NAC is also given for Tylenol/acetaminophen overdose. There is some research suggesting NAC benefits people with autism as well as people with obsessive-compulsive and other psychiatric conditions, which share some symptoms with autism spectrum conditions.
- Magnesium—helps with hundreds of the body's processes and can have calming effects.
- Selenium—is important in detoxification pathways.

- Molybdenum—is important in detoxification pathways.
- Zinc—participates in at least two hundred chemical reactions in the body, and is often abnormally low in autism.
- B vitamins, including B_1, B_2, B_3, and B_6—help facilitate biochemical reactions especially as part of mitochondrial energy production.
- Cod liver oil—is a tried-and-true source of essential fatty acids and vitamins A and D. Read the labels carefully to see if the product has been filtered for contaminants.
- Fat-soluble vitamins A and E—can be low in children with gut problems and poor absorption.
- Vitamin A—is important for fighting infection and for color vision.
- Vitamin D—This vitamin (which some think should be called a hormone) plays a myriad of other roles in addition to bone health, as indicated by a growing body of research, including helping with DNA repair, supporting the immune system, and boosting the production of glutathione. Federal guidelines are based on research on bone health but not much on the other roles of vitamin D, since at present more research is needed on these other functions.
- Folinic acid—a variant of folic acid that is important in pathways related to DNA and methylation.

Food Sources of Nutrients

Ana drinks a juice called MonaVie, made of fruits of a whole spectrum of colors and designed to contain a wide variety of antioxidants and phytonutrients. She says she tried to switch to a less expensive source of antioxidants—a 4–6 week supply of MonaVie costs about $130 in the United States—but it wasn't as helpful. Without MonaVie, she says, her energy level "falls off a cliff." This treatment appears to be biologically plausible and low risk, but expensive. Alternatives that also supply lots of phytonutrients include fruit and green smoothies, but it would be hard (and more expensive) to buy enough fresh produce to replicate the large range of plant species that are included in this one drink. Powders also are available, but research to judge which is better is not likely to come soon.

A rainbow-colored diet with lots of fruits and vegetables of many hues is ideal and something to strive for whether you're drinking a product like this or not. It's much harder to overdo vitamins and minerals if you get them from food rather than supplements.

A rainbow diet rich in phytonutrients has added benefits. Involving your child in picking out and handling these fruits and vegetables can help build perception, skills, and relationships over time.

Cruciferous vegetables are particularly good for helping the body make glutathione. These include broccoli, kale, collard greens, cauliflower, and more. We all know that these are not favorites with children, but with a VitaMix you can start getting small amounts of these into your child, mixed in with other more tasty veggies and other foods. Some children learn to love these veggies. Broccoli sprouts are especially high in sulforaphane, which is the ingredient in cruciferous veggies that helps with glutathione production.

If you're trying to figure out how to get as many antioxidants as possible, you may hear about ORAC, or Oxygen Radical Absorbance Capacity. This is a laboratory test that rates foods for their antioxidant capacity. It's a good rough estimate, although it has not been demonstrated to correlate with health benefit, and food producers can't put it on food packages.

Electromagnetic Frequencies

Ana experienced discomfort around electromagnetic frequency exposure, and she and her doctor felt that the most toxic part of her current environment was electromagnetic radiation from the computers around her at work. This is an area of significant controversy but there is some evidence of adverse effects, especially in children, of problems from exposure to electronics, such as cellphones. There are concerns that these technologies could alter the electrical and magnetic properties of cells, which are important to how cells signal and to how they maintain chemical differences between what is inside and outside their cell membranes.

Ana uses a negative ion generator to combat the positive ions created by electrical equipment. She also sits in an office chair stuffed with magnets to help absorb radiation. She says both help her feel better and more energetic. "I find it impossible to work at my office job in a large office building without them," she says.

I do not have a solid evidence basis for evaluating these products so cannot recommend them. But I do feel that you should be alert for research that may emerge on electromagnetic frequency exposure.

Detox

You may notice that even though I talk about cells and detoxification, Ana did not undergo any explicit detox regimen, such as chelation. Why is that? Ana's doctor believes that the body has its own natural detoxification capacities and that the best way to eliminate toxins is to strengthen the body's own detox equipment. I basically agree, but not everyone does.

There are three issues here: 1) Is there really any toxic body burden in the first place, and if so, does it matter? 2) Do the body's detoxification processes really need help? 3) If so, is helping them with good nutrition and other natural support enough? On all three of these, medical evidence is thin and controversy is substantial.

1. *Is there really any excess toxic body burden in autism?* Blood tests have not necessarily supported the existence of excessive levels of toxins in people with autism. However, blood levels tell you only about recent exposures. They don't tell you much about toxins that may have gone to hide in tissues like bone or fat. I think we need large-scale systematic studies with carefully chosen measures to really understand what the range of toxic problems may be in people with autism spectrum conditions.

2. *Do detox processes really need help?* Medical experts often say that our detox processes work fine on their own and you don't have to worry about it. I don't think there's enough research to say that with confidence, particularly about people, such as those with autism, who may already have genetic, immune, nutritional, and metabolic vulnerabilities and a history of prior exposures. I think medical science needs to investigate this idea more thoroughly. In the meantime I think it is prudent to follow the advice I am giving throughout this book to avoid toxic

exposures and eat nutrient-dense foods that maximize the body's health and resiliency.

3. *Is it enough to help these detox processes with good nutrition and other natural support?* I think there is no substitute for good nutrition. Parents who may wish to go further than this have two options: a) various natural products that can bind to toxins in the body, and flush them out; b) trying chemical aids to detoxify the body. There is surprisingly little research on the effectiveness of medical approaches to eliminate toxins; most research has focused on prevention rather than treatment.

There is some research to support the effectiveness of various natural products in binding to and removing toxins and heavy metals from the body. These products include chlorella (an algae), modified citrus pectin (from citrus fruit), sodium alginate (a common food ingredient made from seaweed that is also sold as a supplement), and cilantro (an herb from the supermarket that can also be purchased as an extract). These are often recommended together with use of fiber products such as ground psyllium seeds (available sweetened in most drugstores or unsweetened in specialty stores) or activated charcoal to keep toxins from being reabsorbed in the intestines. These products have not to my knowledge been tested specifically in autism. They all carry several risks:

1. In binding to toxins they can also bind to vital minerals and carry those out of the body, too, depleting important nutrients;
2. Because they have a chemical affinity for toxins they may absorb toxic substances during production. This means these products could be giving your child extra toxins, rather than removing ones that are already prsent.
3. Even if your child has excellent communication skills you may not get a direct report of any discomfort or complications. In very sensitive children (which includes many with autism) these include problems like an increased stress response, which you may not realize is related to the detox process.

I would discourage this approach unless you have close medical monitoring and support from an exceedingly competent, trained medical professional, as well as lab data on the quality of the products you are using, to confirm that they are not contaminated. Even if you are consulting a well-trained or certified clinician, I would urge you to be extremely cautious if you pursue this.

If you are determined to push this issue further, you should think very seriously about the following issues:

1. Deaths from chelation have been reported. According to the U.S. Centers for Disease Control and Prevention, these have been due to medication errors. Without the assistance of a very well-trained practitioner, you may be putting your child at serious risk from errors in treatment.

2. Attempting detox without first getting all other systems in good shape is likely to make your child worse. Nutrition and gut function in particular need to be in excellent shape before detoxifying. Chelation removes minerals vital to life and health, and mineral status needs to be rigorously monitored and maintained during treatment. If your child is having trouble absorbing nutrients, it is not the time to put the vital mineral supply at further risk.

3. Chelation agents are more aggressive than natural treatments in pulling toxins out of places where they are "hiding." If these toxins are not thoroughly and rapidly excreted from the body, there is great risk of their landing somewhere else and harming another organ, such as the brain, kidney, or heart. If your child's digestive system is not working optimally this is a particular risk. For example, if your child is constipated and the stool filled with toxins stalls out in the intestines, the toxins could be reabsorbed, causing new harm.

4. Standard medical practice is to use chelation for cases of extreme poisoning, but it does not support the use of it for less severe or chronic levels of toxicity.

The bottom line is that at present there is very little research to determine the role of toxicity in autism spectrum conditions, and the safety and effectiveness of chelation is still in question.

It makes sense to take a medical risk on a lifesaving treatment like chemotherapy for cancer, but until there is more solid research on toxicity and its treatment in autism, my own recommendation is to avoid toxic exposures, maximize nutritional support for natural detoxification systems, and avoid unnecessarily risky medical treatments.

In the next chapter, I will walk you through how these same factors—genes, food, bugs, toxins, and stress—affect the organ systems of someone with autism, creating more vicious circles that can exacerbate problems.

KEEP IN MIND

- Cells are basic to everything we do.
- Cellular energy is very important to everything we do as well.
- Most problems in autism are not unique to autism; it's the sum and interaction of all of them, and the age when they start, that create the autism.
- There are many things that can go wrong in mitochondria and other cell functions.
- Cell problems with different causes can cause similar health issues.
- Cells do better when they get good care and feeding.
- Take a systematic approach and keep track of what you do and what happens.

But also remember

- Cellular problems aren't always the first link in the chain.
- Not everyone with autism has mitochondrial problems.
- Cell problems can be hidden or subtle; they may not be obvious.
- There isn't any single, common cellular problem that's the same in everybody with autism.
- Chelation therapy is risky and benefits for autism are unproven.
- Cellular health changes over time, and how you support it may need to change, too.

CHAPTER 4

Get Gut and Immune Systems on Your Side

Long before the autism diagnosis, the discovery of genetic problems, or the celiac disease, there was the diarrhea. For as long as Nell Kubik and her husband, Eric, can remember, their daughter Crystal had runny stools—often a half-dozen times a day. Her poop was always incredibly foul-smelling and so acidic that they had to change Crystal's diaper immediately or she'd develop painful blisters.

At a specialist's suggestion, they tried cutting back on the fruits and vegetables she loved so much—too much fiber was her problem, the doctor said. That helped a bit with frequency but did nothing about the stench, the acidity, or the consistency, Nell said.

Her doctors repeatedly told her there was no connection between her daughter's autism and gut problems. But she's confident there is. If there weren't, why did she learn so much more about her daughter's digestive system from other parents at the special needs preschool than from that gastroenterologist?

Those other parents eventually convinced Nell to bring Crystal to Dr. Ali Carine, a board-certified osteopathic pediatrician in Ohio. After a few visits and some tests, Dr. Carine diagnosed Crystal with celiac disease, a disorder in which the body reacts to the protein gluten—found in bread, pasta, most cereals, and other grain products—as if it were an invading army. Crystal started on a gluten-free diet in early July, shortly after turning three and a half. Within days she "became increasingly verbal, not as emotionally fragile," her mother said. She stopped flapping her arms and was generally more comfortable, Nell said.

But it still took five full months before Crystal, now four, had the first fully formed stool of her life. Nell says she's pretty certain it was the gluten that made the difference, because they avoided making other changes during that time.

Crystal isn't much in touch with how her body feels—even what it's like to feel the need to poop or to actually go. So Nell was shocked recently when Crystal started saying, "I am pooping!"—and she was. Now her parents hope to have her out of diapers by age five.

Also over the past few months, perhaps because of the diet or because of the sensory work she's doing at preschool, Crystal seems to have figured out how to chew properly. Before, she might have taken one bite out of a hot dog and then tried to shove the rest of it into her mouth, often choking. Now, Nell says, Crystal understands how to take regular bites and chew one before taking another.

In addition to her autism and celiac, Crystal has a genetic disorder called isodicentric chromosome 15. That means she has an extra chromosome 15, just as people with Down syndrome have a third chromosome 21. So many people with idic(15), as it is often called, have autism that it is sometimes considered an "autism gene," though most people with autism have an unaffected chromosome 15, and not everyone with idic(15) has autism.

There's no way to change Crystal's genes. She's stuck with that extra piece of genetic material, which can cause mental retardation, developmental delays, and such weak muscle tone that walking is difficult. Crystal's symptoms are relatively mild, but as her mother says, she will always have some problems.

And yet Crystal is doing much better now than she was. Just as every medical symptom shouldn't be blamed on autism, having a genetic diagnosis is not a life sentence, it's just one part of the web.

Nell says she's a show-me-the-evidence type who never thought she'd set foot in the offices of an "alternative medicine" doctor. But now she's completely convinced of the power of dietary changes and biomedical treatments. "Dr. Carine calls me her 'really?' mom," Nell says, chuckling. "Every time she tells me to do something I look at her with a raised eyebrow and say 'Really?' I tell her to her face, 'You are crazy.' But everything she has told me to try has been right. And it's not just placebo effect because people who don't know we're trying it notice a difference. It's not just me hoping."

The Autism Bone Is Connected to the Digestive Bone and the Immune Bone

Digestive problems and immune issues are so often seen in autism that it's reasonable to make a connection between the two. The science isn't conclusive yet, but we're getting there.

As with Crystal's celiac, many parents and clinicians observe that autism symptoms seem more severe when gut or allergy problems are worse. Brain, immune, and digestive problems probably all trigger one another. Feeding, digestion, and/or absorption problems keep the body and brain from getting the supply of nutrients they need to grow, to make repairs, and to do their metabolic jobs. Allergies and autoimmunity may irritate an already vulnerable brain, and they waste energy and resources by attacking "enemies" that aren't really dangerous. A poorly nourished body with a distracted immune system is more susceptible to infections that can drain its resources further. At its worst this is another vicious circle.

But like all of our other vicious circles, the good news is that once you can see it, you also see opportunities to intervene and help. To do this you need to identify leverage points in the web. That is the journey I'd like you to follow me on now.

DIGESTIVE SYSTEM

Gastrointestinal Distress

No one knows precisely how many people with autism also have gut problems. Estimates range from a low of 9 percent to a high of 91 percent. Some years ago, when one doctor announced on the radio that there was no connection between autism and digestive problems, word is his mailbox was quickly deluged with dozens of diarrhea-filled diapers to teach him a lesson.

Until recently, most of these gastrointestinal problems either were dismissed as unrelated to autism and therefore unimportant, or were attributed to "the autism" and therefore considered lifelong, hopeless, and untreatable. In late 2009, a panel of pediatric gastroenterologists, allergists, autism experts, and others, led by Dr. Timothy Buie, a colleague of mine at Massachusetts General Hospital, concluded that digestive problems are real in autism and should be treated as they would be in any other patient. The panel, which published its findings in the prestigious journal *Pediatrics,* also determined that behavioral problems in people with autism are often the result of gastrointestinal pain. Diagnosing stomach pain in someone with autism can be challenging, though, according to the panel, because he or she may not have the vocabulary to explain what's wrong, or, like Crystal, the self-awareness to understand where it hurts.

Food allergies can also be a major source of gastrointestinal distress, the panel found, potentially causing pain, diarrhea, vomiting, behavior problems, gas, and canker sores, among other symptoms. Skin and breathing problems can also be related to gastrointestinal issues.

RESEARCH SPOTLIGHT: GASTROINTESTINAL-AUTISM CONNECTION

Researchers at Vanderbilt University and Massachusetts General Hospital looked at the digestive health of 918 people from 214 families touched by autism, including parents, siblings, and affected kids.

The results, published in the journal *Pediatrics*, showed that 41 percent of those on the spectrum had gastrointestinal issues, compared with 24 percent of their parents, and 9 percent of their non-autistic siblings.

Statistical analysis showed that this breakdown would have happened by chance only 1.5 times in a trillion, meaning the connection between autism and gastrointestinal issues is real. If anything, at least some of the parents underreported problems—rather than imagining their child's misfortune and inflating the numbers.

Many GI problems may also be in the "gray zone"—they may not meet the criteria of a formal disease diagnosis, even though they are bothersome. These ailments are sometimes hard to measure, too.

From Stem to Stern

The gastrointestinal system is basically a long tube for processing food. It works best when each section along the way does a thorough job. People with autism may have hang-ups at every step, which can snowball into big problems lower down. Let's take a tour of the system:

Mouth

The mouth is not just where food is taken in and tasted, but also an important first workstation in digestion. Chewing breaks down food and allows it to mix thoroughly with saliva. This starts the chemical breakdown of large molecules into small ones that can be absorbed. Many people with autism are very picky eaters, rejecting certain textures and tastes, refusing some foods and craving others. Some of this has to do with sensory issues and some may be related to allergies and food sensitivities. Anatomical issues in the mouth might also be involved in digestive issues. If a person has misaligned teeth, trouble chewing and swallowing may follow, which puts an extra strain on the digestive system. Autistic children often have trouble sitting in dental chairs for proper cleanings, orthodontia, or to fill cavities. If teeth hurt, children will avoid eating. When little Crystal took crazy bites and didn't chew her food properly, she was sending down big lumps of food unprepared for the next steps of digestion.

The mouth, of course, also does double duty as our organ of speech. A baby who has trouble with organizing biting, chewing, and swallowing may develop into a toddler who has trouble producing clear speech. Claudia Morris, a physician and researcher at Children's Hospital of Oakland Research Institute, in California, found that nutritional problems are behind many cases of verbal dyspraxia, speech problems such as difficulty with pronunciation, use of words, and understandable speech. She published results of a survey in which 187 children with dyspraxia were given vitamin E and polyunsaturated fatty acid supplements. Ninety-seven percent of the families who responded reported dramatic improvements in speech, imitation, coordination, eye contact, behavior, sensory issues, and development of pain sensation. Morris wants to test whether deficiencies—particularly of the fat-soluble vitamins A, D, E, and K, omega 3, zinc, iron, B vitamins, and amino acids—may contribute to speech problems.

Esophagus

Resuming our tour down the GI tract, we enter the esophagus, a hallway-like tube between the entry point of the mouth and the major workstation in the stomach. Rates of reflux, in which food and stomach acids come back up the esophagus, seems to be astoundingly high in autism. In one study of thirty-six children with autism, researchers from the University of Maryland found that 70 percent had reflux, compared to 2 percent of kids with neurotypical development. Reflux can be painful and can cause sleep problems and lead to behavioral outbursts—as it did for nearly all of the children in the Maryland study. Allergies can also trigger irritation of the esophagus, as can poorly chewed food. Once the lining of the esophagus is eroded, it is more easily inflamed, feeding the vicious cycle of pain and deterioration. Pain from cuts in the esophagus can turn children off to eating and may be a major trigger both for aggression and for self-injurious behaviors like head banging and self-biting.

Stomach

In the stomach, enzymes break down food and acids kill or inhibit dangerous bacteria that was in the food. The stomach also sends signals to the brain about the nutrients it's getting, to ensure the body gets what it needs. Lots of things can go wrong here: Enzymes fail to completely break down food (many kids seem to do better when they take a digestive enzyme at the start of a meal); stomach acids may be weak or in poor supply, allowing dangerous bacteria to survive; or poor chewing may leave chunks of food untouched by enzymes or acids.

Small Intestine

The task of the small intestine is to break down larger molecules into smaller ones and to absorb nutrients from the gut into the bloodstream. Food is absorbed through the villi, tiny fingers that line the walls of the intestines and serve as a link between the digestive system, the blood-stream, and the immune system. You can see why it is a good idea to do the best possible job at the mouth and stomach workstations, because food that reaches this point without having been properly processed is too large to be absorbed by the villi.

Diseases like celiac, as the family of four-year-old Crystal discovered, can damage the villi, making it harder or nearly impossible for the intestines to absorb nutrients. According to extensive research by Alessio Fasano at the University of Maryland, gluten causes the release of the protein zonulin, which opens the gaps between cells in the lining of the gut wall, making more room for things to pass through. While this happens in everyone, in people without autoimmune disease the gap closes right away. But in people with an autoimmune disease—including celiac, diabetes, multiple sclerosis, rheumatoid arthritis, many psychiatric illnesses, and possibly autism—this gap stays open for an extended period of time and closes very slowly. While it is open, gluten and other foreign substances (including bacteria and viruses) can get into the bloodstream and trigger an immune response. As the immune response snowballs, it wears down the gut wall's villi and stresses other parts of the body, including the brain. Removing gluten from the diet can interrupt this cascading process. Children with autism whose villi are damaged by gluten often show dramatic improvements when gluten is removed from their diets, though, as with Crystal, it usually takes months for the villi to repair themselves.

Many people also give up casein, a key protein in milk, in order to get rid of digestive and emotional symptoms.

Although the gluten-free, casein-free (GFCF) diet is considered controversial, by now there are a number of good-quality scientific studies supporting its efficacy. In one carefully designed large study, the children who were supposed to be in the control arm, keeping their regular diet, were taken off gluten and casein midway through because the children on the diet had done so well. These studies are hard to conduct because it's so tough for everyone to eat the same way when they're choosing their own food, and also because some of the gluten- and casein-free substitute foods are of poor quality and may cause their own problems. See examples in the help section below.

Other parts of the gut lining may also cause problems. Mucous membranes are supposed to smooth the food's journey and help protect the gut. But if the cells that generate the mucus aren't functioning properly, the food may not slide so well through the gut and the gut wall may not be properly protected. Sulfur is needed to make the mucous lining and if there are problems with sulfur, that may contribute to weaker gut linings, as well.

The last part of the small intestine, the ileum, is the only part that can absorb vitamin B_{12}, which is critical to brain, blood, and metabolism. If the ileum is inflamed or overgrown with bacteria, it will be hard to absorb vitamin B_{12} from food. This vitamin cannot be obtained in a vegetarian diet without supplementation.

Large Intestine

Nearing the end of our tour of the intestines, we come to the large intestine, or colon. Here water is absorbed, but not much food apart from some vitamins and minerals such as potassium. Undigested food fiber and food fragments are fermented here with the help of gut microbes. If fermentation doesn't go well, though—if the bugs are wrong and/or the food hasn't been properly processed to this point—the result can be nasty gas and the foul-smelling stool that led one group of autism parents to nickname themselves Poops-R-Us.

Sometimes mostly digested food gets stuck at this point. Hard stools can jam the system, leading to painful constipation. When stool is impacted, watery diarrhea may pass around the edges, masking the problem. Diets that lack fiber can lead to constipation, as can the milk-heavy diets common among people with autism. Sensory problems, like Crystal's, can make it hard for children to know when they need to use the toilet.

Sometimes the problem is: a digestive system slowed down by a virus, a lethargic thyroid, the side effect of medications, or chronic stress. Slow transit time, which may be due to weak "peristalsis"—the waves of gut wall muscle activity that move the food along down the digestive tract—can also be related to weakened mitochondrial energy.

Got Bugs?

One of the biggest scientific revolutions in digestive system research is gut bugs. This world of billions of tiny organisms in your intestines is now as scientifically exciting as the genome was ten or fifteen years ago. Gut microbes play a huge role in the intestines. "Good" bacteria help us break down and metabolize food, but modern life often conspires against these helpful bugs. Antibiotics wipe out the bad bacteria that may have triggered an infection, as well as the good ones that help with digestion. Once demolished, the good bacteria may be replaced by opportunistic ones—almost like weeds that take over your garden faster than the flowers you planted. These opportunistic bacteria may also anchor themselves in a "biofilm" layer along the gut wall, cleverly hiding from the immune system.

Numerous research studies show differences in gut bugs according to where you live, what you eat, and what diseases you have. Illness can be associated with "dysbiosis"—which means a problem with gut bugs. Small bowel overgrowth—lots of nasty bugs in the small intestine—can interfere with absorption of vital nutrients. People who move from one part of the world to another will swap out their gut bugs and get colonized by gut bugs in their new home locale. Jeff Gordon of Washington University in St. Louis has shown that obesity may be caused in part by gut bugs that change your metabolism when they colonize your intestines. This produces excess calories that are transformed into pounds. Changing what you eat can change your gut bugs in as short a time as a single day.

Gut bacteria can also affect your brain. More and more studies are showing that gut bugs can lead to mood changes and other psychiatric problems. Feeding depressed people fructose or lots of carbs can make their symptoms worse, and this may be due to changes in gut bugs.

Some studies suggest that abnormal gut bugs may play a role in autism, although more research needs to be done. These include abnormal types of bacteria, such as clostridia, and abnormal chemicals that bacteria can make. Chemicals from gut bugs can affect the brain. Gut bugs can also steal nutrients from us by chowing them down themselves, and spitting out toxic trash that goes upstairs to the brain and makes trouble. In 2011, Antonio M. Persico and colleagues reported that the urine of young autistic children contained a chemical called p-cresol. The more the p-cresol, the more severe the autistic symptoms, they found. This chemical is not produced by human metabolism, but by gut bugs—

it's absorbed into the bloodstream and then excreted by the kidneys. Gut bugs are consuming the sulfur that ought to be going into the children's bodies to support their critical sulfur metabolism. We already know that children with autism often have problems with sulfur metabolism from their own genetic vulnerabilities and from toxic exposures; gut bug chemicals can make it worse. Even more sinister, this chemical can disrupt mitochondrial function by interfering with the production of ATP, the cell's energy source.

RESEARCH SPOTLIGHT: GUT BUG RESEARCH IN AUTISM

Jeremy Nicholson's research group at Imperial College, London, found different chemicals in urine from autistic than from unaffected children. These chemicals were made by an abnormal species of gut bacteria, clostridia.

After finding abnormal clostridial bacteria variants in the stool of autistic children, Sydney Finegold of UCLA's David Geffen School of Medicine and the U.S. Department of Veterans Affairs found that children with autism showed short-term improvement when taking vancomycin but got worse again after stopping the antibiotic. When taken by mouth this high-powered antibiotic is not absorbed but kills clostridial bacteria in the gut—but not clostridial spores, which may have grown back more bacteria after the antibiotic was stopped.

Researching mice, Derrick MacFabe at the University of Western Ontario measured the impact of chemicals produced by gut bacteria on the brain and on behavior. The symptoms were similar to those seen in autism.

The eating habits of autistic people can compound the problem of abnormal microbes. A low-nutrient-density, high-energy diet—in other words, starchy or sugary junk food—provides lots of fuel for the nasty bacteria but not much nutrition for the person. It may be that some of the dramatic results people report from diet change in autism (and other conditions) comes from gut bug regime change—starving out the nasties and supporting those that promote health.

IMMUNE SYSTEM

Protecting the Borders

While we can tour the digestive system from top to bottom, the immune system is structured more like the federal immigration service. It has agents all across the country, but they are especially concentrated at the borders, the interfaces between the inside and the outside—including the gut, lungs, and skin. The immune system is not just about defense against enemies, though. It also plays a critical role in information sensing, communication, and regulation.

The immune system is particularly active in the digestive tract. Gut-associated lymphoid tissue, or GALT, includes the tonsils as well as the lymph tissues in the intestines and appendix and comprises the largest portion of the body's lymph tissues. Some of the lymph tissues' other hubs include the lungs, skin, nose, tonsils, salivary glands, larynx, and eyes—all of which come into direct contact with the outside world. Then there's the bone marrow, the spleen, and the thymus, which produce, educate, and process immune cells.

The immune system is constantly interacting with the environment—and with the gut and its bugs; its knowledge base is greatly shaped by these interactions. Babies need experiences to develop a robust immune system.

Human immune systems evolved to cope with a world that most of us no longer know. The "hygiene hypothesis" argues that modern people are so sanitary, we no longer get as many exposures to dirt and bugs as our ancestors did. Those exposures educated our immune system. On the other hand our immune systems are currently getting both educated and miseducated through exposure to all kinds of experiences never before available: new kinds of foods, new chemicals, new germs, new sources of radiation, new forms of social environment—and new combinations of gut bugs, too.

Educating Immune Warriors

Though we have lots of hints, it's still not clear when the immune systems of people with autism start veering off a "normal" course—it may not be the same for everyone. What we do know is that everyone's immune system experience starts before birth, before conception even. The health and immune status of the parents, especially the mother, contributes to the education of a child's immune system. Parents with an autoimmune disease—such as diabetes, rheumatoid arthritis, or celiac—run a higher-than-average risk of having a child with autism. And a pregnant (or soon-to-be-pregnant) woman's allergies, infections, and toxic exposures can all affect her fetus, though we are just beginning to understand how this happens.

Several researchers have shown that immune or infectious conditions during pregnancy can change the baseline settings of the immune system, making the body more vulnerable to neuropsychiatric conditions like autism and schizophrenia. Several studies have found that a number of mothers whose children went on to develop autism showed some indication of immune problems during pregnancy. But we still don't know how strong an influence these immune problems might be, whether they are enough by themselves to "cause" autism, and if not, then how many other genetic vulnerabilities or environmental triggers need to accumulate to push a baby or toddler toward autism.

With birth comes a whole range of new exposures: breathing, eating, medications, vaccines, gut microbes, stress—all contributing to the education of the immune system. The moment of birth may be crucial, too. Because the uterus is sterile, infants have no gut bacteria until they get exposed to them during delivery. In one 2010 study, a University of Puerto Rico researcher showed that babies who are born by C-section and therefore don't go down the birth canal get a different range of gut bacteria than infants delivered vaginally. Among ten newborns, the four born by vaginal delivery had the same range of gut bacteria as was found in the birth canal, while the six born by C-section had bacteria commonly found on their mother's skin, not gut. Scientists are just tooling up to really explore the health implications of these differences.

During the earliest days of life, whatever bugs are present in the baby's gut establish themselves as what the body considers normal. This foundation of familiarity and expectation lasts a lifetime—if the bugs are shifted, as by antibiotics or illness, they tend to drift back. There appears to be a particularly short window for laying down this baseline—possibly just the first month of life, most likely a lot less than the first year. If this familiar baseline is healthy, that will benefit the child, perhaps forever. If the infant or the delivering mother has problems that require antibiotics, the balance of bacteria in the gut is markedly changed, and if the balance is not restored during this early window, the baseline may create predisposition to allergy or other immune problems. Preliminary research is suggesting that giving probiotics to the mother during pregnancy or breastfeeding and to the baby during this first month may reduce the amount of allergic disease that baby will have down the road—but it will take a while for researchers to figure out whether there are specific strains or combinations of bacteria that help the most.

Plenty of people without autism suffer from similar allergic and immune imbalances—perhaps for some of the same environmental reasons. We don't yet know why some get autism, others asthma or diabetes, and still others remain healthy.

Too Much, Too Little, Too What?

Immune problems in autism may vary from person to person. They can be divided into three basic categories: an over-response, an under-response, and a confused response. Allergies are an overreaction to an otherwise harmless substance like ragweed or peanuts. Trouble fighting infections is an under-response. And chronic inflammation and auto-immune problems are what I call confused responses.

In healthy people, there is a balance between two arms of the immune system. One arm, called Th1, deals with infections that invade the cell. The other arm, called Th2, generates an allergic response and copes with bacteria and other invaders that are outside the cell. Health suffers with the loss of this immune balance. It's common for people with autism to have a reduced response to potentially dangerous infections (that is, less Th1), and hypersensitivity to things that may not actually be harmful (that is, more Th2). It's almost as if allergies distract the immune system, leaving it short on soldiers to battle infectious invaders.

Allergies can also deplete coenyzme Q10, an important mitochondrial nutrient, as well as glutathione. This is bad for mitochondria and may contribute to low energy problems and oxidative stress.

Chronic inflammation may also be more common in autism. Inflammation is a normal response to an injury or infection, marshaling the special resources the body needs to fight off an immediate danger and heal tissues. But in many of us, inflammation has become a way of life. It doesn't know how to quit. Chronic inflammation is confusing for the cells, and can trigger obesity, heart disease, cancer, diabetes, and autoimmune problems. It can trigger swelling of the lymphoid tissue in the gut, the nose, the skin, the lungs, the eustachian tubes (which drain the middle ear into the throat), and elsewhere. This can make you feel sick and it can provide stagnant places where infections can breed.

Let's look, for example, at what can happen to the ears with inflammation. Swelling of the tissues lining the eustachian tubes can trap fluid in the middle ear. Just as a summertime puddle becomes a breeding ground for mosquitoes, so this pool of liquid attracts viruses or bacteria that can cause infection. (Next time you see a baby lying down and drinking from a bottle, remember that this can allow milk to back up in the drainage canals.) A healthy child can probably fight off an infection unaided; something like 90 percent of ear infections clear up on their own without medication. But a child with a reduced Th1 function may need help fighting back. An antibiotic may help clear the infection (if it was caused by bacteria and not viruses), but it also knocks down good bacteria in the gut, and doesn't treat the cause of the initial swelling in the lymph tissue, so it's likely that the infection will return. This is another one of our vicious circles.

RESEARCH SPOTLIGHT: INFLAMMATION STIMULATION

Autistic children also seem to have too many immune substances called "pro-inflammatory" cytokines, and too few "anti-inflammatory" cytokines. Research led by Paul Ashwood at the MIND Institute at the University of California, Davis suggests that children with autism have a different profile of cytokines than neurotypical children, with more of the pro-inflammatory variety. Those with the most pro-inflammatory cytokines, his research finds, are most likely to have a regressive form of autism and most likely to have behavior problems. If he and his colleagues are right, this suggests two key things: Immune problems can lead directly to behavior problems, and regressive autism might potentially be a sign of an immune disorder. In a 2008 study, the UC Davis researchers found that children with autism have lower levels of blood immunoglobulin—an antibody that protects against bacterial and viral infections—compared to children with developmental delays and those with typical development. The less immunoglobulin in the children's blood, the more behavioral problems they had, the researchers found.

Crystal's Inflammation Transformation

Recently, Crystal caught a bad cold and her coughing was ruining her sleep. Dr. Carine didn't want to put Crystal on antibiotics, so instead she prescribed a short course of prednisone, a steroid used to treat inflammatory conditions.

For those five days, Nell says it was as if she had a different child. Crystal talked nonstop. "I thought her head was going to explode" from talking so much, Nell said. Crystal chattered about the winter-themed gels on the dining room window. About how polar bears are white and like snow. About how the other gels were brightly colored . . . And she said things that no one had told her to say, which she had never done before. "It made sense. It was spontaneous. It was commenting on her environment in intense detail. There was more eye contact, more engagement. It was like she was a part of the world," Nell said.

Unfortunately, those gains disappeared with the last of the prednisone—as Dr. Carine had warned that they would. Prednisone is simply not a medication that should be taken for an extended period. But both Dr. Carine and Nell got a glimpse of what Crystal's brain can do when it's not inflamed. This is yet another story of a higher-functioning brain being "in there" but obstructed.

Dr. Carine recently tripled Crystal's daily dose of curcumin, hoping to create the same anti-inflammatory response as they saw with the prednisone, but without the same risk. Curcumin is made of turmeric, the bright yellow spice related to ginger that has been used as an herbal remedy for centuries. It is now being studied as a possible treatment for cancer and Alzheimer's disease, because it has promising antioxidant and anti-inflammatory powers. It's too soon to know how Crystal will react to it.

WHAT YOU CAN DO

Gastrointestinal and immune issues affect many everyday choices. Here's what you can do about food, toxins, bugs, and stress to promote healthier immune and digestive systems.

Food

Stick to high-quality food.
Caleb, from chapter 1, made great gains when his mother changed the family's diet to all organic and got rid of all processed foods and food additives. Whatever else you do, it's important to emphasize high-nutrient-density foods—lots of fruits and vegetables—and avoid simple carbohydrates like white bread and crackers, and junk, like many or most packaged foods, and candy. Your child's immune system really needs all the high-quality antioxidants and phytonutrients it can get.

Add gut and immune symptoms to your food diary.
Now that you're focused on food issues, go back to the food diary I suggested in chapter 2 and include more detail about gut and immune problems alongside your other observations. Look for patterns. Do you notice more tantrums, irritability, or sleep problems when your child eats certain foods? What about foods he or she seems to crave? Food addictions and cravings are often signs of hidden allergies. Are there behaviors associated with the times when cravings crop up?

Even if you don't see obvious gastrointestinal problems, they may still be there. Sometimes the only signs are irritability, nighttime waking, unexplained tantrums, refusing to eat, head banging, self-injurious behavior, or a child repeatedly putting pressure on his/her abdomen.

Tests to Discuss with Your Doctor

Nutritionist Assessment

It's a good idea to get a basic nutrition evaluation, looking at growth curves for weight, height, and head size for age, and for basic nutritional adequacy.

Allergy Testing

Skin testing is the most sensitive, but it is not always practical. So-called RAST (radioallergosorbent) testing is less sensitive, but because it involves analyzing blood rather than eating the food, it makes sense if you suspect a dangerous allergy. RAST tests don't catch everything, though. If your child's test is negative but you still suspect digestive problems, getting a serum immunoglobulin G_4 level may be useful.

Elimination Diet and Food Challenge Test for Allergies

An elimination diet and food challenge is probably the best way to reveal food allergies. It is generally done under medical supervision, although if you're trying only one or two foods you might try it on your own. If you're eliminating more than a few food items at a time, get a doctor or nutritionist involved to avoid nutritional deficiencies during the testing. It's important that you completely eliminate the suspected foods during the trial. You need to read food labels and ask questions at restaurants, to make sure they don't sneak items in as hidden ingredients. You also need to be suspicious of ingredients that don't give you specific information: For example, "modified vegetable protein," which appears on many packaged foods, doesn't say where the protein comes from and often the sources are allergenic, such as gluten or soy.

Celiac Testing

Screening for celiac disease may include blood tests for nutritional, immune, and genetic markers of risk. Although many doctors might not recommend a gluten-free diet until celiac disease has been clearly established by an invasive test, I personally would err on the side of caution and try to reduce the risk before symptoms advance that far. (If the child has celiac, parents and other family members are likely to have it, too, and might consider getting tested.)

Intestinal Permeability Testing

The lactulose-mannitol test checks for intestinal permeability, the intestinal wall's ability to serve as a barrier to incompletely processed food (as well as bacteria and viruses). While the term "leaky gut" has been greatly misused and many people don't take it seriously, there is published evidence that people with autism are much more likely to have gut permeability problems than the general population. According to one recent study, nearly 37 percent of children with autism were found to have increased intestinal permeability compared to just under 5 percent of neurotypical children. When these children were put on a gluten-free diet, their intestinal permeability went down to close to normal levels.

Interestingly, more than 20 percent of parents of the children with autism were also found to have gut permeability problems.

Full Gastrointestinal Workup

Last but absolutely not least, if your child's GI problems don't clear up altogether with reasonable interventions, or if they are serious when you start, you may want to seek a full gastrointestinal workup. Sometimes problems are garden-variety that go away with better diet, but sometimes a child may have ulcerations, infections, or even parasites that need to be identified and addressed directly. Thanks to the Autism Treatment Network and to the recent American Academy of Pediatrics consensus statement on gastrointestinal problems in autism, it is starting to get easier to find a pediatric gastroenterologist who will perform this assessment on your child with autism.

Diet

Be Concerned About Self-Restricted Diets

Many children with autism will refuse to eat certain foods and crave others. The "beige diet," consisting almost entirely of wheat and dairy, is popular. One friend's son lived for years on almost nothing but saltine crackers and sour cream; his parents were thrilled when they got him to add fish sticks to his repertoire, but of course those are mainly bread and fat, too. This is not a healthy diet.

Diet Matters

As Crystal's story demonstrates, as well as that of Caleb, Ana Todd, and thousands upon thousands of others, changing a child's diet can have a profound impact on autism symptoms. It doesn't work for everyone, but in autism nothing does. There are some sound studies and scientific reasons for taking this approach seriously, because when it does work it can speed gains substantially.

If you try a diet and it does not work there are four possible reasons:

1. It wasn't the right diet for your child;
2. You didn't pursue it rigorously enough;
3. You didn't stick with it long enough; or
4. It was a good idea but you hadn't eliminated other allergens or troublesome foods that were sabotaging the effect.

Remember that the same goes for research studies—any slips in dietary rigor or persistence may make the study results unreliable or meaningless. A good study of the effects of gluten and casein should have subjects eat a diet that is completely free of these proteins in any form for at least three to six months—the longer the better—before rechallenging.

Diet is still a controversial topic in autism but I predict that this will change. In attention deficit/hyperactivity disorder (ADHD), diet is hitting the mainstream. A recent paper in *The Lancet* showed behavior improved for children on a restricted elimination diet, and the authors stated that "a strictly supervised restricted elimination diet is a valuable instrument to assess whether ADHD is induced by food." And of course, the impact of a particular diet may be different from one person to the next.

As with Caleb, many families do not see dramatic differences while they try a diet and only realize that change has occurred after they reintroduce the foods and see deterioration. Then they look back and realize their child had gradually improved over weeks or months. If you try a serious diet change for a while, you may notice that rigidity gets more flexible and short fuses get longer. Just those two things could make life and learning a lot easier.

Avoid Sugar

I cannot say it often enough. Sugar is junk food. Evidence suggests that not only does it feed bad bugs but it can drive inattention, impulsiveness, and inappropriate silliness; promote inflammation; reduce resistance to infection; and play into all manner of other behavioral, learning, and health complications. It's just plain bad for cell health.

Wheat and Dairy, Gluten and Casein (and Starches!)

The gluten-free, casein-free (GFCF) diet tops the popularity list in helping to reduce the symptoms of autism. GFCFSF (SF is soy-free) is popular, too. As I have already mentioned, there is scientific research on neurological, autoimmune, and other health problems that can occur with all of them. When someone who has derived the majority of their calories from wheat and dairy stops eating these foods, they can go through withdrawal, like an addict coming off drugs. I had a two-year-old patient whose parents had started him on this diet before seeing me. He had done well on GFCF for two weeks—he started making eye contact, and babbling when he hadn't talked, and his skin rashes went away. But then he abruptly lost all of his gains. His family had no idea why, since they were being strict with his food, until they found him crawling on the floor stealing the cat kibble—which was loaded with wheat and dairy.

Some families go "cold turkey" to get it over with all at once. They may prepare and transition the whole family over to this diet, which is easier since the child is not tempted by forbidden foods in the house, and it often makes everyone else healthier, too. Others do better by slowly phasing gluten and casein out of one meal (such as breakfast each day) and then waiting a few days before cutting it from lunches, and then dinners.

This diet can be safe provided the foods your child *does* eat are varied and balanced. Orienting your diet around a high-nutrient-density rainbow diet, or caveman diet approach (eating foods that a caveman could have obtained, such as unprocessed meat, vegetables, fruit, and fish but not cultivated grains, sugars, or processed foods) will help you achieve your goals *and* stay away from processed junk food. It helps you to look forward to the foods that are good for you rather than looking backward at the old unhealthy foods that you miss. You can get support for this diet from a knowledgeable practitioner (doctor or nutritionist) or from books and support groups, but look for a solid commitment to a high-nutrient-density, plant-based diet with unprocessed meat products.

Whatever you do, don't replace gluten with junky "gluten-free" alternatives. If replacements are high in sugar and refined starches of low nutrient density and heavily processed, they are still junk food. These could even make your child's gut bug problems worse. Some gluten-free products might be okay now and then, but breaking the cookie and sandwich habit is even better—that way, your child won't be tempted to cheat, and you won't have problems like Crystal did when her grandmother accidentally fed her bread she thought was gluten-free. (Crystal gobbled down three slices and then spent the evening in the emergency room having seizures that may have been triggered by the gluten.)

Keep the gluten and casein out of the diet for a period of time. In the case of gluten it takes three to four months to get it out of the system and to allow the gut wall to repair itself. If you see a clear improvement (or if your child cheats and falls apart, which in and of itself is a sign that something was working before the regression) there is no reason to try to reintroduce gluten anytime soon. If you try a food challenge, reintroduce a small amount of a specific food to see what happens. Track this carefully in your log. Notice your child's behavior, sleep patterns, and any change in his or her digestive system. Sometimes deterioration is not immediate but takes place over some weeks.

Milk is a whole different story. A brief review of the problems with milk is in a little book called *Don't Drink Your Milk,* by the late Dr. Frank Oski, author of *Oski's Pediatrics.* He argued that most people simply are not designed to drink milk after early childhood. Oski also discussed the fact that all cows aren't created equal. Fifty or sixty years ago the milk Americans drank came from small, light brown Guernsey or Jersey cows. Then farmers switched to the larger, black-and-white Holstein cows because they had bigger udders that were easier to milk. But milk from Friesians (Holsteins) is chemically different, with less protein, less calcium, and fewer omega-3 fatty acids than milk from Guernseys or

Jerseys. It is also high in a different type of casein that is more likely to cause allergies.

Cows are also fed antibiotics, and their grain-based—rather than grass-based—diet may deplete the vitamins in milk, and may cause food sensitivities. To boot, when milk is pasteurized, some good bacteria is cleared out along with the bad.

Diet: Specific Carbohydrate Diet

This diet eliminates starches and not just gluten. It is targeted at the gut bugs that like to chow down on sugars. Some people who fail the GFCF diet do much better taking this further step. (See the "Bugs" section below for more details.)

Other Diet Sensitivities

Don't overlook the possibility that your child is sensitive or allergic to something totally unexpected or weird. It was only after her child had been on a gluten-free, casein-free diet for some months that a mom I know realized her son had an intolerance for corn, too. Some parents report that their child's poop-smearing habit stops after they eliminate corn. Other kids have trouble digesting soy. And some can't handle the oxalic acid found naturally in foods like spinach, kale, and almonds. Their bodies can't seem to break down the acid, and the crystals that form can irritate the bowel and lead to intestinal permeability.

My friend whose son couldn't tolerate corn told me that although she's a scientist by training, she feels like she has to be Sherlock Holmes when hunting for guilty foods. It's about trial and error and really observing, she told me. When her son's karate teacher would praise his focus or how in control of himself he was in class, she'd consider what he'd been eating over the last two to three days. When his behavior slipped, she'd do the same. When she saw red cheeks, red ears, dilated pupils, or dark circles under his eyes, she knew he'd eaten something he shouldn't have. Regardless of what food he ate, his face and skin responded the same way. But interestingly, different foods triggered different behaviors. Corn made him wet his bed, she told me. "He would pee gallons, two to three times a night. Blue food dye did the same thing; whereas red food dye was like wheat."

After several years of a specific diet, some food sensitivities can go away, so you may consider retesting every few years to see if you can re-introduce the food.

Grass-Fed Meat

Cows evolved to eat grass, not grain. Grain (like corn) gives them what we might call "heartburn" and gas. This is treated with antibiotics to "help them grow," which they probably need because their gut bugs are messed up from the grains. About three-fourths of American antibiotic production is used in animal agriculture, and when animals poop it out, these antibiotics get into our water supply. These practices have been banned in much of Europe. Grain feeding of animals also requires a lot of petroleum-based pesticides and chemical fertilizers, which are a problem in our current economy; they cause pollution and deplete vital soil minerals. Grain-fed meats come from animals that are usually also treated with lots of antibiotics and hormones. You can ask for grass-fed meat at your supermarket and you can also go to your local farmer's market, and sign up for regular orders of locally grown grass-fed meat. It is more expensive, but generally of much better quality.

Picky Eater Strategies

If your child is an extremely picky eater with a very restricted diet, be suspicious: There's likely to be a problem underlying such strong food preferences—gut issues, allergies, or dental difficulties. Time to put on your Sherlock Holmes hat and take data on everything. Fussiness could be a sign of nutritional weakness or indicate allergies or food addictions. Try broadening his or her range. If texture is an issue, keep experimenting until you find a more diverse list of nutritious foods. Zinc, which is found in meats, dairy, beans, and pumpkin seeds and as an over-the-counter supplement, can help improve the function of taste buds and get kids more interested in new foods. Behavioral training can also help children accept new foods (I'll address this in chapter 7).

Digestive Enzymes

Many children seem to do better if they take a digestive enzyme capsule at the start of a meal; clinical trials are presently under way to see if this observation holds up scientifically. Outcomes may be complicated by differences in which specific enzymes children may need to be supplemented.

If you are following an elimination diet like GFCF, a digestive enzyme is not a substitute for rigor. Just because you're using an enzyme that targets problem foods, don't think you can reintroduce the off-limits foods without consequences.

Immune-Supportive Supplements

In addition to curcumin, which helps calm down a lot of inflammation pathways, some other supplements important to immune health are fish oil (omega-3 fatty acids), vitamin D, vitamin A, and zinc. All of these can be dosed too low or too high, so get trained supervision here.

The bottom line is that there's a lot of guesswork, experimentation, and inconvenience involved in changing a child's diet—but there are some clear, basic principles, and the payoff is potentially huge.

After the large gain Crystal saw from removing wheat, her attempts to get rid of dairy have been rockier. She still has enough autism symptoms that her doctor wanted her to try going without dairy, but a month or two after she went casein-free, her behavior and health deteriorated abruptly. She had a bout of pneumonia, and she seemed to get more and more "autistic" as time went on, her mother, Nell, said. About three months later Crystal's parents began reintroducing dairy.

Toxins

Your child is likely to be a lot more sensitive to the effects of toxins than the "average" person, so it's important to play it supersafe. Once someone is sensitive and vulnerable, further exposures increase the risk of what Claudia Miller of the University of Texas Health Science Center at San Antonio calls "Toxicant-Induced Loss of Tolerance," or TILT. Put simply, the more reactions your immune system has, the more reactive it can get. Here are some recommendations for what you can do:

Avoid pesticides by eating organic as much as possible.

If you can afford it, organic foods are preferable to conventionally grown ones, particularly fruits and vegetables where the skin is eaten. Pesticide residues are not good for your child's health, behavior, or brain.

Dirty Dozen (highest in pesticides; buy these organic if possible)

Apples	Grapes (imported)
Celery	Sweet bell peppers
Strawberries	Potatoes
Peaches	Blueberries (domestic)
Spinach	Lettuce
Nectarines (imported)	Kale/collard greens

Clean Fifteen (lowest in pesticides)

Onions	Cantaloupes (domestic)
Sweet corn	Kiwis
Pineapples	Cabbages
Avocados	Watermelons
Asparagus	Sweet potatoes
Sweet peas	Grapefruits
Mangos	Mushrooms
Eggplants	

Source: Environmental Working Group, www.foodnews.org/executive.php

Avoid meat containing hormones and antibiotics.
Your child may be delicately balanced in the systems that are impacted by the hormones and antibiotics given to conventionally raised animals. Better to seek out products that don't contain these. Food markets that sell organic products may carry them. Grass-fed meat from organic farmers will generally also be hormone- and antibiotic-free.

Avoid excitotoxins like MSG and aspartame, used in
    NutraSweet and Equal.
I think it's wise and important to avoid excitotoxins in food, particularly aspartame and MSG. These chemical additives feed into the oxidative stress cycle to which your child may be particularly vulnerable. They can especially drive brain problems that I will tell you about in the next chapter.

Avoid artificial ingredients, food additives, and food dyes.
After years of assurances that food dyes were safe, solid research is now showing a clear impact on developmentally vulnerable children exposed to food dyes; Europe is moving to strict labeling policies and there is discussion about it in the United States. Try tracking your child's behavior carefully in your food diary and look hard for the little things, like the impact of the food dyes in the free lollipop from the bank that you might forget to write down. One of food guru Michael Pollan's basic rules is to avoid foods with ingredients you wouldn't cook with yourself. If there's no xanthan gum in your kitchen cabinet, there shouldn't be any in your dinner, either. Another rule of thumb you can use is "don't eat anything you can't pronounce"—if it's a long, complicated chemical name, have a really good reason for eating it or skip it.

Avoid big fish.
Big fish eat smaller fish and thereby concentrate toxins in their bodies. Tuna and other large fish—the highest on the food chain—are especially high in mercury and other toxins. Mercury is an immunotoxin and can worsen any autoimmune tendencies that may exist. In one experiment with mice, Ellen Silbergeld and colleagues at Johns Hopkins University found that the equivalent of as little as one can of tuna per week was enough to worsen lupus symptoms. Even low concentrations of mercury affect the immune system by throwing off cytokine signaling pathways, they said, potentially making people more susceptible to infectious or autoimmune diseases.

One handy rule of thumb when shopping for fish in the grocery store is that if you can see the mouth and tail of the fish, it's a small fish. If you see a circular piece with the backbone on top and steak-like slabs of meat on left and right, this was a sideways slice through a big, long fish.

Bugs

Starve out the "bad bugs."
Avoid simple sugars and starchy carbohydrates that feed unhealthy bugs and contribute to persistent abnormal gut bug ecology. For the most part, they are also low in vital nutrients and in fiber. Avoid starchier varieties of beans like chickpeas (also called garbanzo beans).

The Specific Carbohydrate Diet, which avoids all starchy carbohydrates, was originally developed for people with ulcerative colitis and Crohn's. It uses nut flours in place of grains. It allows home-cultured yogurt and honey, but some with autism may not tolerate the dairy and may have "bad gut bugs" that adore the honey. Some of its recipes may usefully expand a caveman or rainbow diet.

Support the "good bugs."

Nondigestible fiber is abundant in vegetables and legumes (beans). Our guts are designed for a high-fiber diet. This fiber is fermented into products that support healthy immune function. On the other hand, diets low in healthy fiber promote the growth of unhealthy bacteria like clostridia.

Learn about fermented and cultured foods.

Naturally fermented foods, such as sauerkraut, kefir, cider, many cheeses, and "real" sourdough breads, are excellent sources of probiotic organisms to keep your gut bug population healthy. Nearly every culture has a tradition of eating fermented foods. Factory-produced foods are largely made without fermentation, because the process would add to the cost.

Probiotics

Although studies are not completely consistent, data is accumulating that probiotics can help build a healthy immune system. Although eating them in food is ideal, taking them as powders mixed in food or drink or in capsules can help build up a struggling digestive system. But beware of sweetened yogurts, like those marketed to children. The sugars added to the yogurt feed the bad bugs and counteract the probiotic, rendering it useless. It's much better to eat plain yogurt with fresh berries or in a smoothie.

Probiotic supplements can be helpful if they're taken during or right after antibiotic or other treatments that kill gut bugs. All by themselves probiotics have not been shown to permanently fix the gut ecology, perhaps because they don't contain other substances that would come along with them if they were part of a food. They work better if they are supported by a high-nutrient-density, high-fiber diet. In its latest report on probiotics, in December 2010, the American Academy of Pediatrics finds probiotics safe for all children except those who are seriously immunocompromised or chronically ill. Though more research is still needed, the report concludes that probiotics are at least moderately effective at treating stomach viruses in healthy children and in preventing antibiotic-associated diarrhea in healthy children. They may also have a positive benefit for irritable bowel syndrome, chronic ulcerative colitis, and infantile colic, but not for cancer or Crohn's, according to the report.

Homeopathy

Some of the patients you'll read about in this book, including Caleb and Ana, say they have seen benefits from homeopathic remedies.

Homeopathics are meant to stimulate the body, particularly the immune system, to react to things including chronic infections so that it can relearn how to react appropriately. It's based on the idea that the body can learn to cope with a lot of something if it is primed with a little first. Most scientists dismiss homeopathic medicine, saying it is not plausible that such heavily diluted treatments could do anything (though many homeopathic treatments are not heavily diluted).

Before you pursue these treatments, you should know that while these remedies are for the most part low risk and have a low to moderate cost, their efficacy is not well supported, and the philosophy and training of practitioners can vary widely.

Track infections in your log.

Make sure you note infections and fevers in your log along with food, sleep, behavior, and other things. Infections can interact with the immune system, metabolism, toxins, and energy production in complicated ways. If you see patterns, they may provide useful clues for you or your doctor about what might be causing or complicating your child's autism and possibly what might help.

Vaccinations

Vaccination is one of the most powerful protections against the scourge of dangerous infectious diseases, such as polio, measles, and meningitis.

They are the best protection we have. Their effectiveness relies upon the participation of the vast majority of the population, so vaccination is about both protecting your own health and protecting the health of society.

We are also learning that infection is influenced not only by the bug you caught but also by your state of health. That means that how serious your infection gets is influenced by your genes, your metabolism, your immune system, your toxic exposures, and your gut bugs—as well as by how well you eat, how much you sleep, and how stressed you are.

In this light, how do we make sense of the concerns some parents have that their child may be fragile and vulnerable and may have a hard time with vaccines? Some parents say that their child stopped talking and started showing autistic behaviors shortly after a vaccine. This could be a coincidence, considering that symptoms of autism often first appear between ages one and two, when shots just happen to be most frequent; or it could be a sign of a genetic, metabolic, or immune vulnerability.

With the giant strides being made in molecular genetics and immunology, we are beginning to learn about individual differences that may put people at higher risk of having adverse vaccine reactions. Researchers at the Mayo Clinic in Rochester, Minnesota, are developing new scientific fields with names like vaccinomics (the development of personalized vaccines) and adversomics (the study of the genetic and immune basis of adverse vaccine reactions). With the knowledge these fields generate, we may eventually be able to design science-based accommodations that protect vulnerable people from dangerous infectious diseases in ways that work best for them.

In the meantime, we need to do our best with what is available to us now. I strongly encourage vaccination. That said, we need more data on how children who have autism and perhaps other known or unseen vulnerabilities respond to the current vaccination protocol.

To address concerns you may have about vaccines when your child gets vaccinated, you can apply the strategies I have been suggesting throughout this book: Build your child's strengths, and remove or compensate for your child's risks. Provide the best possible, high-nutrient-density food, avoid health-depleting junk food and toxic exposures— these are fundamental to helping your child's immune system respond the way it should. So are avoiding exposures to allergens and keeping your child's gut healthy.

I also suggest that if your child is in the middle of an illness, infection, or fever, reschedule your vaccine appointment and get the shots when your child is well again. I think it is also prudent to request preservative-free vaccines, from single-dose vials if possible, and to avoid giving too many vaccines at one time. If your child has missed some shots because of illness or scheduling problems, think twice before doubling up on shots. Instead make another appointment, even though it may mean another copay.

You may wish to consider giving your child extra antioxidants, N-acetylcysteine (which helps make glutathione), essential fatty acids, and probiotics over the days prior to vaccinations to boost their immune system. It may be better to use ibuprofen (e.g., Motrin, Advil) rather than acetaminophen (e.g., Tylenol) if your child develops a fever after the shots, as acetaminophen has been shown to lower glutathione levels, potentially increasing immune vulnerability and oxidative stress.

If you have questions or concerns, please talk them over with your child's doctor. While I understand the importance of a rigorous vaccine schedule, I believe that getting vaccines stretched out over a longer time is far better than not getting them at all.

Stress

Stress is hard on everything. The fight-or-flight stress response diverts blood flow away from digestion and slows the peristalsis muscle activity that moves food through the gut. Stress also challenges the immune system, promoting inflammation and reducing resistance to infection. These are already likely to be big problems for your child, so managing stress effectively is important for immune system health.

My main advice here—which I know is easier said than done—is to look for ways to make eating fun rather than stressful. One mom I know got her son to help her make vegetable smoothies. He still refuses to drink the smoothies, whose texture makes him gag, but in touching the vegetables, he got intrigued by them and began to take bites. Now he's eating peppers and cucumbers and a range of vegetables he never would have tried before. Cooking with children is one of the great joys of parenthood—particularly on the weekends, when you're not in a rush and can handle the extra mess. Don't deprive your child or yourself of that pleasure. At minimum, it's good quality time together. At best, it helps build independence and encourages your child to try new foods.

In the next chapter I'll show you how genes, food, toxins, bugs, and stress can change the way the brain functions.

KEEP IN MIND

- The immune system and digestion play a huge role in autism.
- An explosion of science supports a gut-immune-brain connection.
- Gut bugs are more important than we ever imagined to both health and disease.
- Food and nutrition can make a really big difference to the autism web.

But also remember

- There is no one-way causal chain between the gut and the brain or the immune system and the brain.
- Not everybody has the same gut or immune problems.
- Vaccinations protect against diseases that can be very dangerous.

CHAPTER 5

Help the Body Mend the Brain

An eleven-year-old boy with autism speaks in longer sentences when he runs a fever. "Where he might usually use three or four words, he was using six or seven" during a recent illness, his mother says. On a more typical day, he might say, "Mommy, Tinker Bell," when he wants her to put on his favorite movie. While sick, it was, "Mommy, I want to watch the whole Tinker Bell."

A father from Boston tells a similar story about his four-year-old son. When sick, the boy uses multiple, complex sentences that he doesn't use when he's well. After the fever fades, many of the improvements do, too. His mother taught him his numbers during a recent illness; the figures stayed past his return to health, but his use of complex sentences disappeared.

Similarly, the O'Leary family can go months without hearing an understandable word from six-year-old Jo, until she has a fever. Once, she spiked a temperature of 105.9 and the thermometer hovered around 104 for a few days. She suddenly sang the words to the *Teletubbies* theme song (her favorite show) and belted out the *Bob the Builder* song with sounds like words. For about a month after that last fever, her communication skills progressed—she correctly labeled animals and said and used more words appropriately. Eventually, though, as after previous fevers, she regressed and stopped talking again.

"What we took away from [the last fever]," her mother, Katherine

O'Leary, said, "was the knowledge that the words were actually in there somewhere."

Listening to Parents

For years, parents had been considered crazy when they said their child seemed to emerge from autism during a fever. New language was considered a fluke, a coincidence, or the parents' imagination—after all, it went away again after the fever subsided.

But Laura K. Curran and her colleagues at the Johns Hopkins Bloomberg School of Public Health in Baltimore decided to take those parents seriously. She examined thirty children with autism and fever, and though it was a small study, she confirmed that the kids showed fewer autism symptoms when feverish. PKU, the disorder that leads to mental retardation if children eat protein, showed us that diet can have a dramatic effect on the brain. So fever and a few other triggers of short-term improvement suggest that the brain is not irrevocably "disordered" by autism. When something like a fever alters the brain, it often seems to work as if there were no autism there at all. We saw the same thing in the last chapter, when little Crystal "became a different child" in her mother's words, while taking prednisone. Some antibiotics also produce temporary improvements in some kids.

I'm not at all suggesting that any of these things should be used to treat autism—because they certainly should not. But the mere fact that they can trigger change in what has been seen as essential parts of "the autism" suggests the brain may not be as hardwired as we thought.

Genes can't explain these rapid changes; your genetic code can't transform itself in a matter of hours. Nor is the brain rearranging its anatomy fast enough to show the changes we see with fever. Instead I suggest—admittedly with just the beginnings of research so far to back me up—that autism may be more of a "state" that can change than a "trait" that is fixed and unchangeable. Change can come very quickly when a blockage is somehow removed or a previously unworkable connection is made. If we can figure out what causes the blockages or how to overcome them, we may find ways to help the brain and the whole person reach their full potential.

A brain that just isn't working right has what doctors call an "encephalopathy." *Cephalo* means "brain," and *pathy* means illness. *Encephalopathy* means "global brain dysfunction."

Medically, autism has long been considered to be a "static encephalopathy"—a kind of brain dysfunction that is not going to change, almost like a birth defect of the brain.

In recent years, more and more neurologists and neuroscientists have decided that it is really more of a "dynamic encephalopathy," because it *does* change: It may be different from day to day, it may get created over time rather than being imprinted from the start, and it may improve or get better.

The Brain Depends on the Body

Remember the last time you were drunk, deliriously tired, or seriously jet-lagged? Your brain probably didn't work as well as it usually does. Maybe you were clumsier than usual, slower to notice things, quicker to forget. Something you did to your body—drinking, flying, or depriving it of sleep—had a profound effect on your brain. I believe the same connection is at play in autism. Something that goes on in the body is limiting the brain's ability to do its job properly. Something that is affecting the body's cells is affecting the brain's cells, too. Autism certainly won't be as easy to fix as skipping a beer or taking a nap, but from a whole-body perspective it makes sense that helping body cell health will improve brain cell health, too.

The human brain performs a huge amount of work. At any given split second, 100 billion of your brain's neurons may be sending signals. All this electrical activity requires a huge amount of energy and lots of supplies. Brain cells need twice as many calories as other cells in the body. The adult brain also burns up 20 percent of the body's oxygen, even though it weighs only a few pounds, and the young brain burns up an even larger percentage of the body's oxygen supply.

This oxygen, as well as nutrients and calories, depends on a well-functioning bloodstream to transport them from the lungs and the gut into the brain.

THE BLOOD-BRAIN BARRIER (BBB)

The brain is protected from many things the blood delivers to other parts of the body by the blood-brain barrier (BBB), an extra layer of protection, because cells can't afford to get sidetracked by infection, inflammation, or toxins.

The BBB separates blood from brain tissue and the fluid in the brain. It helps maintain a stable environment for the brain and keeps out things that don't belong. It is made out of a thin membrane, specialized blood vessel cells, and brain cells called astrocytes that wrap around the capillaries and blood vessels of the brain.

This blood-brain barrier isn't foolproof—meningitis, for instance, is caused by a brain-swelling infection that sneaks through the barrier. And it isn't fully formed until around a child's first birthday; before that, more toxins and germs can get in. Around the base of the brain are several areas where the blood-brain barrier is always more permeable. This gives the brain several windows through which it can "sense" the chemical state of the blood, and gear up to respond to it. If there are toxic agents circulating in the blood, they can enter through these portals, too.

Just as the blood-brain barrier separates the blood from the brain, the gut-blood barrier separates what passes through the gut from the bloodstream. Both barriers can be weakened by everyday or common experiences, such as illness, infection, inflammation, stress and exposure to toxins, microwaves, radiation, injury, trauma, and physical pressure.

Finally, the mitochondria in the brain cells must be healthy and in good working order to produce adequate energy from these supplies and oxygen. If any part of this supply chain or infrastructure isn't working up to par, the extraordinary demand on these cells can run ahead of supplies.

Brain cells are particularly vulnerable because alongside their need for lots of energy, they have low levels of antioxidants to restore damage. The brain is therefore at high risk for oxidative stress.

As you can see, problems with the body—not enough food or oxygen, insufficient vital nutrients, depleted energy resources, damage from toxins or infection—can rapidly cause problems in the brain.

RESEARCH SPOTLIGHT: EVIDENCE FOR MEDICAL PROBLEMS IN THE BRAIN IN AUTISM

Scattered through the peer-reviewed scientific literature are studies suggesting that medical problems with brain energy and supply lines may play a key role in autism. These problems are just the kind you'd expect to come from the interaction between genes and our unhealthy food-, toxin-, bug-, and stress-filled environment. Some autism studies have shown oxidative stress and mitochondrial dysfunction in brain tissue. Almost two dozen other autism studies have shown problems with blood flow and with metabolism of glucose, a sugar.

Examining why children with autism have big brains, a lot of studies show a lower density of cell metabolites, more fluid where there should be more cell fibers, and lower brain activity in the places where these tissue problems occur. Some brain-imaging studies suggest that the extra "stuff" making the brains bigger could be made up of fluid, not cells. It's more evidence that the cells are not working at their best.

These problems with supply lines and energy are also being found in other medical, psychiatric, and neurological diseases. They suggest that the brain is not simply wired differently but is having medical problems.

The Brain's Gray Zone

Depriving the whole brain of oxygen leads to death within minutes. If blood flow is blocked from a particular part of the brain, it leads to a stroke. In other serious diseases, such as Alzheimer's, multiple sclerosis, and other neurodegenerative disorders, vast numbers of brain cells are killed off or damaged.

Luckily we see none of this in autism. With our current clinical tools, we can't diagnose autism with a brain scan. Yet obviously the brain is involved in autism. I suggest that what we see in the brain with autism is another "gray zone"—function that is not "diseased" but not optimal, either. Cells are idling, offline, disorganized, distracted, or sidelined; not dead, but hardly in peak health.

There is growing evidence for this kind of "cell idling" in other conditions, as well. In epilepsy, when neurosurgeons remove a seizure "hot spot," other areas of the brain that had been given up for dead can actually "wake up," according to three separate research papers. It's almost as if once they stopped getting zapped by the seizures, they could pop back up and return to their regular jobs. Toxins can also cause changes in cell electrical signaling even before the cell starts to look abnormal and damaged.

Existing research suggests to me that something similar may be going on in autism, though we don't have studies yet to specifically test this idea. If there were a "gray zone" of reduced (but not absent) function, it would explain how the brain can "pop back" when the autistic person has a fever or takes certain medications. I think these situations show that cells and networks can function better under healthier circumstances. But in their present state, they don't get enough breaks or have the resources to sustain the improvement.

These ideas raise two key questions:

1. Do temporary improvements and the "gray zone" point to explanations for the biology of autism that we haven't considered before?
2. Are there ways we can get these short-term improvements to last longer or not go away?

For the rest of the chapter, I'm going to walk you through the brain's health problems and suggest possible answers to these questions.

MANY DIFFERENT KINDS OF AUTISM

By now everyone agrees that there is no single autism but many "autisms." Not all people with autism may have the kinds of brain problems I am describing here. Although most or all people with autism probably have brain network problems, there may be exceptions.

It is likely that there are many different biological pathways leading to brain network problems. I also suspect that the types of brain cell problems I am talking about in this chapter will prove to be more common than most other brain differences in autism.

Chronic Brain Immune Problems

Aside from energy and supply problems, there is another reason why brain cells might be offline or not at their best: inflammation. As I mentioned in chapter 1, Dr. Carlos Pardo and his colleagues at Johns Hopkins University have spotted changes in the more primitive, "innate" part of the immune system of people with autism. The Hopkins group has also found signs of oxidative stress in the same brain tissue samples, alongside the inflammation.

Once the immune system gets activated, it sets off a vicious circle, too. Pro-inflammatory cytokines can increase oxidative stress, putting cells in harm's way. They can also drive an increase in the inflammation itself, a true "self-amplifying" vicious circle. So oxidative stress and inflammation are deeply related. Inflammation is designed to be temporary, but in the brain, as in the body, it can get stuck. Instead of resolving, it can go on for a long time. Inflammation and other immune distur-

RESEARCH SPOTLIGHT: WHOLE-BODY GENES AND THE BRAIN

Italian researchers Carla Lintas, Roberto Sacco, and Antonio M. Persico recently reviewed gene expression studies in autism and Rett and Down syndromes. In all three conditions, they expected to find a lot of activity in genes controlling early brain development.

To their surprise, they found instead that the shared genes related to more global (and, we might say, whole-body) activities. They concluded that the common pathways among these conditions were an out-of-whack immune response, oxidative stress, and abnormal mitochondrial function.

bances are turning out to be important in brain-related diseases from depression and traumatic brain injury to Alzheimer's and Parkinson's. We are also learning that the immune system plays a critical role not only in brain development but also in day-to-day regulation and signaling, even in healthy people.

Brain Glue

So far, I've been talking about brain cells as if they were one thing. But there are a number of different types of brain cells, and some of the newest research on them may have major implications for autism.

Neuroscientists like to talk about neurons. Even the name of the specialty—*neuro*science—gives that away. For many decades they have studied the electrical pulses and chemical signals that pass across tiny gaps called synapses between neurons. Neurons are the key to rapid long-distance communication in the brain and body.

But as R. Douglas Fields explains in his 2009 book, *The Other Brain*, other cells, called glial cells or glia, make up the vast bulk of the brain—and are turning out to be far more important than we thought. These glia, named for the Greek word for "glue," had been seen mainly as the stuff that kept the neurons in place, like "brain connective tissue," and as helper cells, keeping the neuronal environment clean and well nourished. They were even nicknamed "nurse cells" because of this helper role. But just as we've realized that nurses do far more than keep patients clean and fed (as important as those tasks are), so too are neuroscientists slowly recognizing the many crucial roles played by glial cells.

For our purposes, the important thing is that *glial cells are the interface between the body, brain, and environment.* When we drink too much and our blood alcohol rises and gets into the brain, it is the glial cells that will get drunk first. Glial cells attach to tiny capillaries on one end and feed and clean up after neurons on the other. They are also on the front line of the brain's immune system, the first to get inflamed by cytokines carried in the bloodstream. And they are responsible for regulating neurons. When glia get too stressed and don't do their job right, neurons have trouble controlling how they fire and they can get burned out.

Glial cells are also vulnerable to genetic problems. In the genetic disease Huntington's, for instance, some researchers believe that the single faulty gene that causes the disease acts directly on the glial cells, which then kill the neurons.

I think the glial cells help explain why biomedical approaches sometimes work with autism. The glia perform the functions that are most directly targeted by biomedical approaches. They deal with immune and infectious challenges. They take out the cellular "trash" that will help reduce overstimulation. They control vital metabolic functions, such as supplying the glutathione that is essential for maintaining cell health and limiting oxidative stress. Because they form the blood-brain barrier, they interact directly with the blood system that carries immune messengers. They also play critical roles at the synapses.

Most of the neurons you're born with will also be the ones you die with; very few neurons can regrow. Glia, on the other hand, can regenerate and replace themselves. If you make improvements to food, toxins, bugs, and stress, you have a shot at building healthier generations of new glial cells, improving overall nervous system function.

WHICH COMES FIRST?

Do body problems cause brain problems? Or do brain problems cause body problems? Does the whole body system, including the brain, get impacted at the same time? Or are body and brain problems unrelated? I can imagine plausible ways that each could be true. There is no definitive proof for any one theory. It may be different depending on the person.

Glial Cell Job Descriptions

To help understand exactly what glial cells do, here are job descriptions for the three major kinds.

- The **microglial** cells, the immune system's presidential guard, protect the valuable brain cells. They are normally at rest, but when they sense trouble from bugs, toxins, or stress they get "activated" and start causing oxidative stress and sending out immune chemicals—cytokines and chemokines—that promote inflammation. To defend the brain, the microglia travel to sites of infection, where they gobble up wayward bacteria and viruses, as well as cellular debris.

- The **oligodendrocytes,** which make up about 9 percent of the glial cells, are charged with providing a fatty protective coating called myelin around the fibers (or "axons") that neurons send out to connect to other neurons. This myelin coat insulates the arms and speeds up the signals they carry. The little "oligos" are terribly vulnerable to oxidative stress and can get injured and even die from it. Myelin damage is what causes the symptoms of multiple sclerosis, slowing down and misdirecting nerve impulses.
- The **astrocytes,** which make up as much as 90 percent of the glial cells, are jacks-of-all-trades. As their name suggests, they are star-shaped cells with lots of "points" or processes reaching out to many other cells and to the brain's tiniest blood vessels. They are also the *stars of this story.*

There are three parallel functions of astrocytes. First, as I already said, they play hitherto unsuspected roles in *brain information processing.* They help regulate the neurons' signals by sending signals ("gliotrans-mitters") of their own. They also process sensory information. Astro-cytes talk to other astrocytes in local and giant networks. Many thousands of astrocytes are actually physically connected to one another through little tubes called "gap junctions." A signal starting in one place can set off calcium waves that quickly travel across great distances in the brain. We are learning that astrocyte networks influence the coordination of brain networks—the same networks that research has found have wir-ing problems or "underconnectivity" in autism.

Second, they help maintain the brain's *balance between "excitation" and "inhibition."* Disturbance of this balance may be central to what causes autism. Astrocytes help here by regulating "excitation" or "activa-tion" (stepping on the gas) with a brain chemical called glutamate and providing proper levels of "inhibition" (putting on the brakes) via a chemical called GABA. They do this by mopping up extra glutamate in the synapses and by helping turn glutamate into GABA.

Third, astrocytes *maintain brain health* and are the "trash collectors of the brain," according to researcher Michael Aschner of Vanderbilt University. Liver cells are the trash collectors of the body, and to Aschner, astrocytes are "like liver cells that got lost." They play a critical role in managing the metabolism of neurons, and in helping neurons deal with the oxidative stress they generate with all their electrical signaling.

As part of their health maintenance activities, astrocytes play *protective* roles:

- They are responsible for the neuron's supply of the antioxidant glutathione, which protects the neuron from the oxidative stress "trash" it makes.
- They form part of the blood-brain barrier, which protects the brain from most of the crud that gets into the rest of the body.
- They secrete nerve growth hormones that help build brain connections.
- Astrocytes also mop up toxins, holding on to them and keeping them from doing harm—unless the astrocytes get overloaded.
- Astrocytes play immune roles. They get "activated." Carlos Pardo found activated astrocytes as part of the autism neuroinflammation he discovered.

So, if brain problems are going to be fixed, the glia will do the fixing, and you can support the glia through a nutritious diet, building up the immune system, avoiding toxins, and reducing stress.

NOT JUST THE BRAIN: GLIA IN THE GUT

Amazingly, glial cells have been found in the nervous system of the gut, not just the brain. Michael Gershon of Columbia University showed the interconnection between the nervous system and the gastrointestinal tract in his 1999 book, *The Second Brain*. As in the brain, gut glia outnumber gut neurons by at least 4 to 1, and perform functions much like glia in the brain—they contribute to the gut-blood barrier, they produce immune chemicals, and they help make neurotransmitters, such as serotonin. Though we barely knew they existed a decade ago, we now know that they contribute to conditions involving nervous system or immune dysfunction or degeneration, such as autoimmune disease and diabetes. They also play important roles in inflammatory bowel disease, constipation, and increased gut permeability. To the best of my knowledge, no one has yet studied these gut glia in autism. But I suspect that these cells might have something important to teach us about how gut problems work in autism, what we can do about them, and how glial cells contribute to autism and other conditions.

More Vicious Circles

Here we go again. . . . This whole system works great when it's not stressed. But when it is, there's one mess-up after another.

When astrocytes are overwhelmed by toxins or immune triggers, they swell and start secreting substances that change the brain's cellular environment. They don't mop up as much glutamate. When too much glutamate accumulates in the synapse, the neuron gets overactivated. They fire too much, which requires extra energy from mitochondria, increases the risk of oxidative stress, and can push cells over the edge from functional to dysfunctional. Astrocytes also fall down on the job of balancing glutamate with GABA, and so GABA can no longer calm down the "overactivation."

In addition, the supply lines and trash routes start getting compromised. Swollen astrocytes can squish the tiny capillaries and make them even tinier, limiting the flow of blood that supplies nutrients, antioxidants, and oxygen. Because of the oxidative stress and inflammation that comes with toxins or infection, the blood might become more "viscous" or sticky. And as I mentioned earlier, oxidative stress can also stiffen cell membranes.

Question: How will sticky, stiff blood cells flow through the brain's smallest blood vessels when these tiny capillaries are being squished by swollen astrocytes? Answer: with difficulty. Cellular trash will have more trouble diffusing into the blood vessel to be taken out of the brain. Crud will pile up, causing irritation and interfering with cell machinery.

Meanwhile due to reduced blood flow, mitochondria don't get enough fuel and oxygen, so they can't make enough energy to keep the neurons going.

Researcher Michael Aschner describes these vicious circles as a *brushfire*. "It's going to continue unimpeded," he explained to me. "It feeds on itself." This vicious circle of so-called excitotoxicity and undersupply of antidotes like glutathione and GABA can kill neurons—as we see in cases of stroke and Alzheimer's. But even if it's not bad enough to kill, it can cause persistent problems, putting us right back in our "gray zone."

RESEARCH SPOTLIGHT: BLOOD FLOW IN THE BRAIN

When scientists get pictures of the brain "lighting up" in response to a picture of something or some kind of stimulus, what they are tracking is changes in blood flow and oxygenation. These changes have been interpreted as due to "neuronal activity." But astrocytes and blood vessels are also involved in blood flow. In a review published in 2008, Christopher Moore of the Massachusetts Institute of Technology said the idea that neurons control blood flow and astrocytes is too simple. Instead he presented a large body of evidence for his "hemoneural model," that the neurons, astrocytes, and blood vessels all influence one another. It's not a top-down relationship—all three are interdependent. That leaves us, as you may have guessed by now, with a web.

Coming Unglued—Could This Be the "Ground Zero" of Autism?

In autism, it looks like there is trouble for the whole team. Neurons, astrocytes, and blood vessels are all having a hard time.

In the whole body, it's also not just one thing, but everything: Genes, cells, organs, and brain are all struggling.

In chapter 1, I showed you Caleb's web and said everything was interconnected. Tug on one part of the web and it affects everything else. I also told you that after hearing hundreds of stories from patients, I have come to think that autism is a giant pileup of problems, a buildup of "total load" stretching the web to a point where it doesn't bounce back. Autism lies on the other side of this tipping point.

So what is this tipping point *in the brain*? To find it, we need to be true to the range of stories of people with autism.

- Some people seem born with autism, but we don't know for sure whether it was hardwired into them from conception or built out of an accumulation of problems on top of vulnerabilities starting in the womb.
- Something happens in the brain of a child who was previously functioning close to normal to transform them into someone who acts autistic, even if they were showing subtle signs of dysfunction earlier on.
- Whatever it is that gets in the way of the brain being at its best, for at least some people it is reversible—it can, with a lot of work, get out of the way. Caleb and Ana Todd and Crystal, and all the children who partly "pop out" while they have fever, have brain changes that are not totally fixed and stuck.

The brain can change for the worse—but it can also change for the better. Seeing autism as a web, you can find lots of places to help it shift. And even little shifts can add up to big changes.

How I Think Autism Regression Happens in the Brain:
- Demands are placed on the whole body by some combination of poor food, toxins, bugs, and stress, likely with genetic vulnerabilities in the mix.
- This degrades the support system of the brain—not enough antioxidants, essential fatty acids, and other nutrients.
- Meanwhile the body and brain start to get hypersensitive and overreact with more inflammation and oxidative stress as the problems continue.
- The astrocytes start falling behind in supporting and protecting the neurons.
- The astrocytes and microglia get further distracted by being "activated" as these toxins, bugs, and stressors make bigger demands on the brain.

- This astrocyte and microglia activation produces oxidative stress, which further degrades their function.
- The blood supply to the brain starts declining as sticky blood tries to squeeze through vessels that are constricted by swollen astrocytes.
- When astrocytes can no longer keep neurons calm and balanced, excitation spirals out of control. This increases oxidative stress and reduces the efficiency of mitochondria.
- Astrocytes can't make the glutathione that could bring the oxidative stress down and protect the mitochondria.
- At some point the "total load" is too much, and a tipping point occurs:
  - Astrocyte networks start to fall apart—gap junctions close, communication degrades. Glutamate piles up, making the brain overreact to input from the five senses.
  - Brain networks get weaker and less extensive as cells go into a disorganized, distracted "idling" mode to protect their challenged resources.
  - The brain stops being able to coordinate complicated information processing.
  - In this condition, the brain is overwhelmed and the behaviors it produces look "autistic."
- There are so many vicious circles, each making the other worse. Changing just one thing at a time is unlikely to get this system unstuck. It therefore looks hopeless.

Helping the Whole Brain's Web

The reason I have spent so much effort in this chapter explaining to you about the biology of the brain—about the brain blood flow, energy reserves, neurons, and glia—is that I believe this web represents one of the main roads to better brain function and healing.

If autism were just about neurons with problems, there would not be a lot you could do to address it. Neurons don't regenerate or heal well, and when they die they are usually not replaced.

If the troubles all came from genetic problems with neurons, we would be stuck for a long time waiting for specially targeted drugs and gene therapies to help correct them. And even if a new drug to treat a specific gene problem were developed, if you didn't have the specific gene problem targeted by this drug, you might still be out of luck.

Yet people with autism have been getting better without those precision, high-science interventions. They've been getting better by doing a lot of commonsense, down-to-earth things.

This makes a lot more sense when you realize that your choices can help the brain not only by helping the neurons, but by helping the rest of the brain's web as well.

The Astroglia

Neurons can be helped to send clearer messages by making astrocytes healthier. You can help the astrocytes function better by protecting them from toxic buildup, from immune triggers that "activate" and distract them (avoid those toxins, bugs, and stressors), and by giving them what they need to keep producing glutathione and other vital chemicals (high-quality food and nutrients again!).

The Microglia

The microglia get activated in response to infectious, immune, or toxic stress. Avoiding those toxins, replacing bad gut bugs with health promoting bugs, and reducing other stressors like oxidative stress may well bring balance back to the brain's immune system.

The Blood Supply

You can help the brain's blood supply by improving the quality of what is in the blood (high-quality food!) and helping the blood get less sticky (reducing oxidative stress through high-quality food containing ample antioxidants, and addressing toxin and bug issues).

The Energy Supply

You can support energy reserves by getting rid of the toxins, bugs, and stress that reduce energy production, or by providing nutrients to protect and support the mitochondria.

It's hard for the brain to replace damaged or dead neurons. But glial cells can regenerate, new blood vessels can grow, and mitochondria can be replenished. Restoring the health of these other parts of the brain will support the health of the neurons.

Brain Genes and Environmental Vulnerability

The story I've been telling you about body and brain may or may not involve an underlying gene problem. In some people a faulty gene may be enough to lead to autism. But I suspect that in most of the growing numbers of people with autism, their genes only create vulnerability, and the environment does the rest.

There are certainly genes that could *contribute* to autism. Meanwhile physical problems in the brain can make synapse and network troubles worse. And for most people with autism—those with no known genetic contributors—we have no data on whether these brain and body problems are enough on their own to *cause* autism, or whether they also require genetic risks to turn the brushfire into autism.

Remember Crystal, who turned out to have celiac disease on top of her idic(15) chromosome abnormality? She did considerably better on a gluten-free diet and had an even more dramatic though temporary

RESEARCH SPOTLIGHT: GENES CAN CAUSE ENVIRONMENTAL VULNERABILITY

Researchers at the University of Oklahoma used a simple worm (whose nervous system is easy to work with) to look at neuroligin, which supports the function of synapses. They found that a mutation in the gene for neuroligin triggers oxidative stress.

These same worms also showed sensory processing problems similar to people with autism. And they were more sensitive to the toxic effects of oxidative stress, heavy metals, and the pesticide paraquat.

This is not so surprising. A gene mutation can make a cell more inefficient. Cells that are already genetically teetering on the edge might require less toxic exposure to push them over into dysfunction.

transformation during prednisone treatment for pneumonia. Her story, as well as scientific research, suggests that reducing the physical problems of the brain can reduce the severity of autism even when there is a specific autism gene involved.

WHAT YOU CAN DO

Regluing the Brain by Helping Your Whole Body

If the brain depends on the body, can the body help "reglue" the brain?

There are no scientifically proven treatments for "body problems in the brain" or for reversing blood network problems in the brain. But now you know why I think it makes sense to follow my basic recommendations: These commonsense interventions will create a better milieu in which optimal brain health is most likely.

The Four Essentials—Change What You Can

Food

Perhaps you remember your parents telling you to "eat your brain food." They were right: Food can make a big difference to the brain. Your brain needs loads of antioxidants, phytonutrients, vitamins, and minerals to work at its best. A high-nutrient-density, plant-based diet is by far the best way of securing this solid foundation.

A plant-based diet can also help neutralize acids that could otherwise make astrocytes more prone to problems. I'm not saying that eating a plant-based diet will be a surefire way to directly target your astrocytes. But what I *am* saying is that this diet at least will not put obstacles in the way, and may even help, perhaps a lot.

I already told you in chapter 4 to stay away from excitotoxins (such as MSG and aspartame, as well as hydrolyzed vegetable protein, which usually contains multiple excitotoxins). While some consider it controversial to claim these substances are unsafe, now that you've read about how the brain develops "overexcitation" or "overactivation" when it gets in trouble, why would you want to add fuel to the fire? It's prudent to avoid these chemicals rigorously when you are dealing with a child who already has brain problems.

When your child's brain is this seriously challenged, eating low-quality food like heavily processed food or junk is not optimizing the brain's chance to do its best. Food dyes and other additives are far more likely to add to the harm than promote good, and with your child's brain as fragile as it likely is, adding to the problems is all too easy. Your child cannot afford empty calories.

About 20 percent of the brain is made of DHA, an omega-3 fatty acid that is a prime constituent of fish oil. DHA is incredibly vulnerable to oxidative stress. When your child's brain is in trouble, that fatty acid is likely to be damaged (or "peroxidized") by oxidative stress, reducing the quality of what your child's brain cells can do. The fatty acids can be protected from damage by a high-nutrient-density diet with lots of antioxidants. Abundant healthy fatty acids in the diet can boost the quality of membranes that surround brain cells and mitochondria, making them healthier, more flexible, and less vulnerable to damage. Adding antioxidants and essential fatty acids (through food and additional supplements) helps build healthier brain cell and mitochondrial membranes. Studies show that fish oil supplementation can be associated with better attention, which may reflect these and other underlying brain cell health improvements.

Some things in the brain may change faster than others but all are important. The stickiness of blood may be affected by your last meal. Reducing the stiffness of blood cell membranes through improving the fatty acids in your diet, on the other hand, may take up to three months— the time needed to produce a new generation of blood cells. Astrocyte inflammation may take even longer to address, depending on how much of a genetic, toxic, and/or infectious load is driving it.

But your goal should be to reduce the total load so your child's web can have the best chance of working its way back to health.

One of the earliest nutritional therapies for autism was high-dose vitamin B_6 coupled with magnesium. Research is mixed, though a fair number of studies have suggested that this combination can help a broad swath of people with autism. The treatment also makes some sense biologically. The enzyme GAD_{67} needs vitamin B_6 to turn glutamate into GABA. More GABA means better brakes, limiting overactivation. Vitamin B_6 can be found in foods such as baked potatoes (with the skin), bananas, garbanzo beans, lean chicken and pork, and some fortified cereals. The Food and Nutrition Board of the Institute of Medicine has set an upper tolerable intake level for vitamin B_6 of 100 mg per day for all adults; amounts above that could trigger neurological problems, according to the government panel. However, these neurological problems have only rarely been reported in children who have used this treatment, perhaps because their autism gives them a higher than normal need for the metabolic brain support. Even so, it is a risk to consider and monitor.

Toxins

There are many brain reasons to avoid toxins. Avoiding toxins before and during pregnancy can protect brain development at a particularly vulnerable time. And avoiding toxins all through your life can protect healthy brain function across the life span.

Toxins during pregnancy can change the way a fetus's brain cells grow, find their proper places in the brain, and hook up with one another. Toxic damage can be dramatic, causing major brain malformations. But the effects can also be subtle. A lot of studies show that children exposed to low levels of various toxins during pregnancy have pretty "normal"-looking brains but still show health and intelligence problems, including some loss of IQ points and a higher chance of conditions with learning and behavioral problems such as ADHD and autism.

Some drugs used in pregnancy and childbirth might lead to a child's brain problems. Terbutaline, used to treat lung diseases like asthma and chronic bronchitis and also used to halt preterm labor, has been shown in rats to promote neuroinflammation and to alter the activity of the important brain neurotransmitter serotonin, for instance.

Toxins can also cause direct changes in the brain at any point during life, killing cells or subtly damaging them—pushing them over into one of our "gray zones." This can happen by direct action of a toxin or by triggering or worsening immune reactions or oxidative stress that go on to cause harm.

Toxins like mercury can clearly accumulate in astrocytes, according to Michael Aschner of Vanderbilt, who is an expert in mercury toxicity as well as in astrocytes. This accumulation is probably good in the short run, Aschner told me, because it keeps the bad stuff sequestered inside the cells, protecting the neurons. But "there comes a point where it's too much" and the toxins spill out into the brain. This can set off a vicious circle involving oxidative stress, inflammation, cell changes, and mitochondrial dysfunction.

A Note on Hyperbaric Oxygen Therapy

Hyperbaric oxygen therapy, or HBOT, has been a hot-button topic among doctors and in the press. It is expensive and has very limited scientific support in autism. Some people say it is irrelevant and even dangerous, while others say it transformed their child.

Caleb had forty sessions after several years of other intensive interventions, and at the end of it was ready to go to school. This is interesting but clearly not an argument on its own for HBOT.

Why might HBOT be dangerous? First there is the risk of accidents and fire, particularly if oxygen is being used rather than room air. Second, pressure may damage eardrums or other sensitive tissues. Third, giving oxygen under high pressure may be more than the cells can handle and it could worsen oxidative stress. Yet some animal research suggests that oxidative stress can be lowered by HBOT. Settling which problem will arise (and in whom) requires research.

The United Mitochondrial Disease Foundation says that HBOT is dangerous for children with mitochondrial disease, and some children with autism meet criteria for this diagnosis. Although the 1 in 3 of those with autism who show signs of mitochondrial dysfunction without genetic findings may not be as seriously at risk as children with confirmed mitochondrial disease, and may not be as vulnerable to injury from HBOT, we simply do not have data addressing this.

Some people may say HBOT is irrelevant because autism is a brain condition with genetic but not mitochondrial problems. I disagree with that interpretation of the science. I think that low- or moderate-pressure HBOT has some plausibility for treating "gray zone" mitochondrial dysfunction, where the cells are having a hard time but are not in acute danger, although the few supportive studies so far in autism are not sufficient.

Even so, the devil may be in the details. How do we tell whom it is good for and when it might be dangerous, or what pressure to use, or whether to use oxygen or how much to use? I disagree with people who say that no further research should be done. But I do think that in the meantime this treatment involves many unanswered questions and potential risks. Basically, I don't think we have enough data either to recommend HBOT or to decide for sure that it is always dangerous or useless.

Bugs

INFECTIONS. Bacteria, viruses, and parasites can impact the brain directly, through infections. Some brain infections are quite severe, such as meningitis. If your child ever had a severe brain infection, it could have left some cell changes or scar tissue that could cause irritation or create extra vulnerability.

Toxoplasmosis, for example, is a parasitic infection transmitted by cat feces that, if transmitted during pregnancy, can cause eye damage, jaundice, hearing loss, seizures, and diarrhea in the fetus.

A mother's prenatal infections, if they are bad enough, can also directly impact the brain of the fetus. Even if the infection is milder, like the flu, some studies have shown that the baby's immune settings can be affected and the brain can become more vulnerable to the development of neurodevelopmental conditions such as autism or schizophrenia. It doesn't seem to matter what particular infection the mother had; the impact is driven more by the immune changes after the infection. If the mother happens to be low on glutathione or other protective substances, it's possible that the impact will be greater on her unborn child.

Some bugs soak up and hang on to toxins, which may affect the body's biochemical or immune functions.

GUT BUGS. Gut bugs can also affect how your brain functions. One way is by producing chemicals that cross the blood-brain barrier and essentially act like drugs or in some cases what some people have called "false neurotransmitters." The chemical p-cresol, which Antonio Persico found in the urine of autistic children, interferes with mitochondrial metabolism and could have a significant impact on the brain. Much current psychiatric research is demonstrating that gut bugs have an impact on mood, emotions, and behavior.

Several pharmaceutical companies are intensively working on identifying drug targets based on what we know of autism genetics and molecular neuroscience. They hope to produce medications that could improve symptoms of autism or even reverse it altogether. And they hope to find drugs that have already been safety tested, cutting the time it takes for a federal review and getting them to patients sooner.

If they find a drug that impacts a genetic glitch affecting a lot of people or a lot of molecules that are behaving abnormally in autism, they may be able to help large numbers of people. Given the hundreds of genes, huge potential numbers of environmental contributors, and whole-body complications, it is likely to take more than one drug to create major improvement. Meanwhile you can use the approach I'm recommending in this book—reduce risk and increase support. I believe that this will be worth doing even after drugs for autism are available, because it will clear out obstacles and give the drugs a chance to do their best work.

Stress

I've been defining stress broadly in this book as what happens when demand exceeds supply. But let's go back to the everyday use of the term—being stressed-out. Increasingly scientists are recognizing that such emotional stress can trigger inflammation, in the brain and in the whole body. This works through a hormone called CRH (corticotropin-releasing hormone) and an internal alarm system called the sympathetic nervous system, which controls our flight-fight response. These in turn set off a cascade of responses that suppress the immune system and increase inflammation over time. If stress persists and becomes chronic, the inflammation becomes harder to quiet down.

What this means is that stressors cross levels—emotional stress becomes physical. Remember that it's a two-way street. Physical stress can also become emotional, because an inflamed immune system and lots of adrenaline can make you more emotionally reactive, giving you a "shorter fuse." Think about that the next time your child throws a tantrum. Is it his emotions, his immune system, his neuron–astrocyte–blood vessel interactions, or are these all parts of the same web, facets of the same crystal?

In the next chapter, I will help you explore how the brain's internal activities affect the child you see.

KEEP IN MIND

- The brain is attached to the body.
- The brain needs the body's best support.
- Body health impacts brain health.
- The brain is a physical organ with cells and blood, not just a computer.
- The brain is more than just neurons. It also has glial cells, blood vessels, and other kinds of tissues. All the kinds of cells and tissues in the brain matter.
- Brain cell health is vital to a fully functional brain.

But remember

- My suggested strategies are not scientifically proven ways to target specific problems in your child's brain. But these commonsense interventions will create a better milieu for optimal brain health.
- The biological mechanisms I've described are not the only ones that matter—there are lots more. I've focused on those where there are simple actions that might help.
- These methods don't specifically target the brain or particular brain cells or processes. But they do create a supportive environment that minimizes brain stresses and encourages healthy brain function.

CHAPTER 6

- - - - - - - - - - - - -

Calm Brain Chaos

J immy's head hurt so much, he said it felt like his brain was rocking and shaking. He'd be screaming and he'd vomit, often several times a day. He told his mom he was afraid his head was going to explode. Then five, Jimmy began drawing pictures of his brain, detached from his body and wearing boxing gloves. "My brain is boxing me," he explained.

Shortly thereafter, Jimmy was diagnosed with seizures. His mom, Cindy Franklin, was told he'd probably been having them for a while. Suddenly it all clicked for her. The temper tantrums he'd been having outside restaurants with neon signs might not have been about food after all, she realized. They might instead have been seizures.

For years Jimmy had been a terrible sleeper. He never napped. It would take him two to four hours every night to fall asleep, and the slightest noise or temperature change, or even needing to roll over, would wake him up again for hours. "It was a real good night if he slept four hours," Cindy said. "I was sleep deprived and losing my mind. It was hell."

During the day Jimmy was like a tightly wound spring. He would run up and down the hall, literally for hours. He couldn't sit still.

The tantrums and hyperactivity got Jimmy kicked out of preschool on day two. The letter the school sent home was the first time Cindy had heard the word *autism* outside of the movie *Rain Man*.

- -

Cells Impact Behavior

In the last chapter, I showed you some of the things that might be going on in the brain cells of people with autism. In this chapter I want to zoom out a bit and show you how those vicious circles we saw under a microscope can play out in your home and at school. The brain is at the crossroads between body and behavior, between body and experience. A network of cells trapped in overdrive has real consequences in the real world, leading perhaps to a child who's too wound up to sleep or talk, who's overwhelmed by sensory experiences, whose brain is subject to seizures—and also to a child who can spend hours riding a city bus, poring over a train schedule, memorizing and repeating hotel names, making music, or drawing intricate pictures.

There are seven common dimensions of autism that might be explained by the over- or under-excitation of brain cells I discussed in the last chapter. Those seven dimensions are:

- Sensations and feelings
- Moving through space
- Sleep
- Seizures and epilepsy
- Words and communication
- Intense focus
- Stress

These are not the only possible outcomes from our vicious circles, and there is certainly more going on than I can explain in any one book, but I want you to see the plausible connections between a challenged brain and the types of behavior that make the lives of many parents of autistic children a living hell. The good news is that by addressing the underlying brain challenges, you can make a substantial difference in your child's life (and yours too).

Jimmy still has a few triggers that will send him over the edge. The sound of dogs barking or someone crying continues to trigger sensory meltdowns, making some days at school a real challenge. But as his mother explains, "If he didn't have those reactions to those two things, we would be done." That is, because of changes they've made and ways they've helped Jimmy manage his sensitivities, she wouldn't consider autism a problem for him any longer.

Let's look more closely at these dimensions of autism and what you might do to help your child deal with any that may be a particular problem.

SENSATIONS AND FEELINGS

Sensory Overload

Imagine you are a neuron having a rough day:

- Your astrocyte partners are too busy fighting off an immune challenge to mop up glutamate.
- Too much glutamate means you can't stop sending electrical signals—think of a cartoon character who gets his finger stuck in an electrical outlet and gets shocked over and over.
- Your mitochondria are running out of energy and they're starting to leak electrons that are zapping your membranes, creating oxidative stress.
- Your glutathione supply has run dry, so you can't get rid of those sticky free radicals, or make the zapping stop.
- You are so overwhelmed it's hard to keep track of almost anything.

Now zoom out and imagine that many of the hundreds of millions of neurons in your child's brain are having the same kind of bad day at the same time. Then you, the parent, come along and want your child to pay attention to you. No matter how much he or she wants to pay attention, it's not surprising that that might be impossible.

Now let's zoom halfway back in and imagine you are your child's hearing system. His ears deliver the sound of your voice to his brain, but as I've just described, the brain that receives these signals is in an uproar. What seems to you like a whisper may sound to him like a shout. All the noise is so disturbing that it's hard to make out syllables or words, not to mention meanings. Or, like Ana Todd, the clarity may come and go. Words you speak to this overwhelmed brain don't get processed the way you intended them to. They're just more needle jabs on a bad day. Other senses can be just as overloaded—remember that Caleb couldn't even stand to be touched with his mother's fingertips.

You may be looking at your child with tenderness and kindness as you speak those words. For you that's the natural thing to do. But the emotion in your face adds to the "noise" and stimulation in your child's brain. It's too much for him to track your eyes, mouth, face muscles, sounds, and emotions all at the same time. The signal from every one of these things is intense by itself. It's hard to figure out which one counts most. Your child's brain may know that emotion means something important is happening—but it might be bad, and that's scary. Without an ability to compute the whole picture, the emotion and the expression become hard to look at, even terrifying, so the only solution for your child is to turn his eyes away, to avoid adding more painful intensity.

Are you getting the idea? Your child's sensory universe is likely to be very different from yours. The autistic brain has too much noise drowning out its weakened signals.

This same sensitivity means people with autism can have an incredible eye for light and color, nose for smells, and ear for interesting sounds. They are often drawn to details the rest of us miss, which helps make them such provocative artists.

At the same time they may not link all these details together into a coherent whole (some scientists call this "weak central coherence").

If you don't understand what it's like to live in such an overloaded world, you are likely to think her temper tantrums are "bad behavior," intended to drive you crazy, when perhaps they're really seizures, or just plain overload. If you "get it" that the world to your child feels overwhelmingly intense, you will understand that your child's maddening reactions do make some kind of sense.

What You Can Do to Control Sensory Overload

To increase your child's tolerance of sensations, try to take a whole-body approach to improving cell, body, and brain health. As always, a **multicolored plant-based diet** full of vitamins, minerals, antioxidants, and phytonutrients is critical.

Magnesium insufficiency can be at the root of some hypersensitivity issues. It may be helpful to get levels tested (in red blood cells or cheek cells if possible, because what counts is whether it's getting into cells, not just what's circulating in blood fluids). There is a lot of magnesium in many vegetables, and in a smoothie they will be easier to absorb. Taking magnesium supplements in more than modest doses may lead to diarrhea, so if you use them, spread them out during the day. Epsom salt baths (and rubs), as well as so-called magnesium oil, are ways of getting magnesium into your child's system, allowing him or her to absorb it through the skin and avoiding the diarrhea.

Working with a **sensory integration**–trained occupational therapist can give your child some relief from feeling hammered and disorganized by too many sounds, sights, smells, or tactile experiences. Sensory integration therapy provides systematic approaches to help the nervous system process sensory input in a more organized way. It may involve playful bouncing, brushing, swinging, pressure on the body or joints, and much more. Most children enjoy this kind of therapy and it's a break from some of the therapies that may be more taxing.

A **sensory "diet" at home** can incorporate elements of more calming activities into your daily routine. Some people squeeze trampolines into their backyards, hang swings from doorways or trees, and stock up on scooters, bikes, skateboards, and roller skates. Obviously you need to pick activities that are appropriate and fun for your child.

And don't forget to program **sensory breaks** into your child's school day. Reconnecting with their bodies by jumping, swinging, or simply walking around can ready students to learn.

Pain

Here's a paradox: People with autism often seem to have a huge tolerance for pain, perhaps not even noticing it. Yet at other times they may need a bandage for every little "owie" and won't even tolerate a label in their clothes. The hypersensitivity seems easier to understand. No one knows for sure what the low sensitivity is about. People with autism who put this experience in words may say that they do feel pain, but that they process it differently or feel it at different times.

Jimmy didn't feel pain or have any sensitivity to cold from ages two to seven, according to his mother. When he was two, he pulled a TV off a stand and it hit him on the head. He didn't cry at all. When he got a cut, he would just look at the wound for a few seconds and then return to whatever he was doing. His tolerance for cold water astounded people. When everyone else would be shivering around a pool, he would be splashing and having a good time.

Even if your child can talk, he or she may not be able to tell you about pain. This may be because your child doesn't use language that way (for example, if they are echolalic—just repeating language rather than making words to express their own thoughts). Or it may be because they can't figure out where the pain is coming from, because they experience sensory signals as spread out over large areas of their bodies rather than coming from a single spot.

One day a twelve-year-old autistic boy named Stuart (whose story I will tell in more detail in chapter 9) became unusually peaceful and sweet—he had been having a rough few months, so the change was noticeable. That night his mother felt his forehead and it felt hot. She pressed on his belly. Without changing his tone of voice Stuart said: "Are you trying to kill me?" She took him straight to the emergency room, where they found that his appendix was ten times its normal size and had to come out. But Stuart, though he could talk, had not been able to tell his mother, "My belly is killing me."

A few years ago Judy Endow, an adult with autism (whom you will meet further in the next chapter), started feeling like something was not right. She did not go to her doctor for several days because she did not know what to tell him. All she could identify was that her feet hurt terribly when she climbed the stairs. She finally went to the hospital when it became hard for her to breathe. It turned out she had severe pneumonia and had to be intubated. Her doctor did not understand why it had taken her so long to seek help. It was hard for her to explain to him that her nervous system had not been able to figure out where the discomfort was in her body, and that it had been sending her sensations in places like her feet, far from where her pneumonia was occurring.

Pain Relief
If your child's behavior changes or deteriorates, you should think about looking hard for sources of pain. Is there a chipped tooth, a hidden cut or splinter, an abscess, even a broken bone?

Connecting your child to his/her body can help with appropriate pain sensation. Sensory activities like swinging, spinning, and skin brushing can help, as can getting physical exercise, deep breathing, and doing mind-body activities such as the Feldenkrais Method, yoga, and some slower forms of martial arts. There is scientific support behind the idea that meditation helps with pain relief, too.

You can also help your child get better at identifying the source of pain. When your son hurts his finger, for instance, talk to him about how painful his finger must be and how much better it will feel when you put a bandage or ice on it. The goal is to help your child put words to his experiences (after making sure that that's really what he's feeling). Years of doing this—and it may take years—will help your child pinpoint pain sensations and help the two of you connect.

RESEARCH SPOTLIGHT: INTENSE WORLD

In 2003 researchers John Rubenstein and Michael Merzenich wrote a paper saying that many features of autism, such as sensory, sleep, and seizure issues, could be explained by too much brain excitation and not enough brain inhibition. This was a fresh way of thinking in a field where brain scientists had been focusing on the sizes of different parts of the brain.

In late 2010 researchers Kamila and Henry Markram pushed this further. They described an experiment in which they gave the anti-epileptic drug valproate to rats before birth, and the rats were born with autism-like behaviors and brain wiring. Since animals don't get autism, no animal model is perfect, but they still give us clues we can get in no other way.

The Markrams developed a theory that autistic behaviors are driven by brain changes that make the world overly intense. People with these brain changes are:

- Hyperperceptive of the smallest details of their environment;
- Capable of performing better than neurotypicals on tests of perception;
- Focused on details but not prone to link things into a coherent whole ("weak central coherence");

- Gifted with enhanced memory, particularly for sensory perception;
- Intensely emotionally reactive, with the apparent lack of involvement and interest in the social world being a defense against overload, stress, anxiety, and shutdown;
- Intensively brain reactive, with the capacity to organize sometimes being overwhelmed by intense input, leading to avoidance of new or intense stimulation.

These two models tie together much of the behaviors and neurological features we see in autism. Mark Bear's theory of fragile X has similarities, too. He says that the genetic problem with the brain chemical mGluR5 creates too much sensitivity to environmental change and excessive neural connectivity, protein synthesis, excitability, and excessive body growth. He even noted that the intestines of his experimental animals passed food through too fast.

Although these scientists don't say so, body problems like inflammation and oxidative stress can also contribute to overexcitation, overactivation, and intensity.

MOVING THROUGH SPACE

Clumsy Coordination

Like many kids with autism, Jimmy is also clumsy and has his moments of awkwardness. He used to run with his head pointed downward. "I always said it was like the ground was metal and he had a magnet in his head," his mom says.

Much research suggests that a brain region called the cerebellum, which coordinates automatic activities like walking, plays a role in autism. Carlos Pardo, whom I mentioned in chapters 1 and 5, found more inflammation in the cerebellum than in the other brain areas of autistic children he examined. The cerebellum is also the part of the brain that was particularly large in many small children with autism, according to an earlier, pathbreaking study done at the University of California, San Diego. The cerebellum may be particularly vulnerable to inflammation, oxidative stress, and too much excitation.

Sometimes people with autism can seem like they're in a stupor—staring off into space, oblivious to others around them. The writer Tito Rajarshi Mukhopadhyay, who has autism, talks about how he used to stare into a mirror for hours as a child, completely losing his connection to the outside world. Other people get stuck in a state of overexcitation where they are making seemingly meaningless movements and sounds—sometimes repeating things they've heard over and over. Both of these physical states are labeled "catatonic," though that term is used to describe too many things and may get in the way of observing the great spectrum of activities that are actually going on (which sounds a lot like our overuse of the word *autism*).

Suggestions for Reducing Clumsiness

I strongly encourage you to get your child involved in some kind of **physical activity** or therapy that allows her to gain a better sense of herself in space.

Look for activities that give the experience of rhythm and coordination at an appropriate pace for your child, such as music therapy. Activities that go at a slower place like yoga or tai chi might be easier to follow at first. A good special needs yoga teacher can help get your child started. Aerobic activities that build up a sweat like running and swimming can also lead to reductions of repetitive behaviors. If you start early in organized sports programs, such as municipal soccer leagues, many of the children will be just as uncoordinated as your child, though team sports probably won't work as well past third or fourth grade if your child is still awkward. Many kids with autism are overweight from lack of exercise. Getting them up and moving may also help them reach a healthier weight.

Some children show an amazing gracefulness when **working with animals,** such as horses or dogs, or with plants. Animals are less emotionally demanding than people, and when well trained, can be very calming. Similarly, gardening doesn't feel threatening and can be done slowly. The competence children show here can help them build confidence. Search the Web for animal, pet, equine (horse), or horticultural therapy to find programs near you.

I have also seen children make extraordinary progress with the help of **mind-body practices** like yoga, martial arts, and meditation, and with bodywork such as Feldenkrais, and the Anat Baniel Method, which evolved out of the former. These practices connect brains and bodies with minds and senses, reducing stress and improving feelings of connectedness, strength, and confidence.

Repetitive Movements

Of course another trait common among people with autism is the apparently purposeless, rhythmical, repetitive movement habit, often called "stimming." Jimmy, for instance, bit his nails and hummed incessantly. When he was little, his mom says, he would sit holding an upside-down toy car, spinning the wheels and staring intently. Other children like to hang an arm out the window of a moving car, rock back and forth, flap their arms, twirl their fingers, spin, repeat sounds, stare at fans or lights, smell or lick objects, or do any number of different behaviors. One recent study estimated that 60–70 percent of people with autism perform repetitive movements.

It's unclear what causes these movements. They might be triggered by an area in the middle of the brain, called the basal ganglia, that regulates movement. Or they might be caused by a poor sense of self in space, or gut bugs making chemicals that drug the brain's movement centers. Some research suggests that activities like flapping, rocking, or spinning may also help regulate stress, sensory experience, and pain.

But regardless of what causes them, repetitive movements might not be something you should simply strive to get your child to stop. Indeed they are sometimes described as ways people with autism increase their sensory signal, so they can figure out where their bodies are in space. Try this small exercise to get a better sense of what I mean: Without looking, try to feel your left hand. You probably have some sense of where it is in space, what it's touching, how much your fingers are bent. Now try slowly folding and straightening your fingers. I'll bet you got a clearer mental picture of your hand when you were moving it than when it was still. Some people with autism have a very limited mental picture of their bodies or body parts—this picture may get stronger or weaker during the day. Movements, such as arm flapping, spinning, or swinging, fill in that mental picture to give them that crucial sense of themselves.

As annoying as these repetitive actions may seem, it may be easier to be patient when you understand that they have a purpose. If you look for what's overwhelming the person with autism, or help them fill their sensory needs, they may have less need for these movements. Many children whose parents take a whole-body approach to their autism will stim much less or even stop stimming altogether. Perhaps as their brain and body cells get healthier, the "itch" that the stims are trying to "scratch" gets less and the need to scratch it fades away.

SLEEP

Sleepless in Autism

Sleep is an altered brain state. It changes our "brain waves"—the large-scale electrical rhythms that come from brain cells as they signal together. When we sleep, we damp out signals from the outside and give the brain and body a chance to repair and to integrate new information. After a good night's sleep we are much better able to pay attention, to think well, and to learn. When you haven't slept, things don't go well. You can't think straight. You forget. You make stupid mistakes.

Imagine being sleep deprived on top of having sensory overload problems. Lack of sleep makes it harder to tolerate lots of stimulation. It's kind of like going to a rock concert with a hangover. If you were having trouble with overload in the first place, then sleep deprivation puts your overload in overdrive.

And you can forget about learning. Your mind is pulled in every direction but no one direction enough to get a grip on it. *All the stimulation becomes a source of stress rather than of information.*

About 80 percent of children and adolescents with autism are reported to have sleep problems. Why? Sleep problems can come from too much brain excitation. A brain that can't calm down very well is likely to have trouble sleeping. Brain wave dysfunction can also cause sleep disturbances.

Sleep problems can also come from medical problems, such as gastroesophageal reflux disease, or GERD. GERD hurts and it can wake you up. If your esophagus, or food tube, is already irritated from this stomach acid exposure, the pain itself can keep you awake. Trouble sleeping can also come from other sources of pain.

As you know from your own experience, sleep disturbance can also reduce the immune system's ability to fight off infections. Everyone is more likely to get sick when they're run-down. At the cellular level, what we call *run-down* involves a depletion of the cell's reserves, including antioxidants such as glutathione. Sleep deprivation activates pro-inflammatory immune chemicals (cytokines) that make inflammation worse around the body. In particular, they go to the brain and excite the brain cells.

This brings us, as you've probably guessed, to yet another vicious circle: Poor sleep reduces antioxidants and increases oxidative stress and inflammation, which increases brain excitation, which messes up sleep (as well as everything else that the messed-up sleep already messed up).

Suggestions for a Decent Night's Sleep

There are lots of basic steps for improving sleep. (These are easily found on the Internet by searching for "sleep hygiene.") They include things like: have a regular bedtime routine, limit napping, avoid drinking too much liquid after dinner, don't eat or exercise too close to bedtime, stay away from caffeinated and sugary beverages, avoid foods and drinks with aspartame (Equal or NutraSweet), which can be overstimulating. Limit distractions in the bedroom or sleeping area, turn off or unplug electrical equipment, and block out sources of light.

Getting **regular exercise** every day is also important for promoting sleep—the U.S. government recommends that children get 60 minutes of exercise a day.

For kids with autism it's also important to rule out painful digestive problems that might be interfering with sleep, such as reflux, where stomach acid comes back up the throat. Also look for other sources of **pain**—teeth, bones, cuts, abscesses, splinters—that your child may not tell you about.

Allergies—both food and environmental—can also interfere with sleep. Some allergies can cause hyperactivity, pain, or even bedwetting. (Many people find the same thing with food dyes.) Anyone who suffers from hay fever understands the link between allergies and sleep. Some parents discover that when they eliminate a food allergen such as corn, sleep problems seem to get much milder and bedwetting may go away.

As a toddler, Jimmy was spitting up all the time; he also had terrible diarrhea and flushed cheeks. His doctor said these were all normal, but they went away when Cindy switched his milk to soy. She later confirmed that he was allergic to milk—and, it turned out, to soy as well. His sleep and behavior improved dramatically when she took these foods out of his diet.

Toxins may contribute to hyperactivity, or to grogginess. Try to track your child's exposures in relation to behaviors and sleep.

A warm **Epsom salt bath** before bed helps many children sleep. The magnesium in Epsom salts is a natural tranquilizer, and sulfate can help reduce stress on your child's cellular chemistry. You can make this a part of your bedtime routine.

Melatonin, the hormone that triggers the sleep cycle in all of us, helps many children go to sleep or go back to sleep. It can be given as drops under the tongue or as pills. There is a fair amount of research on melatonin, much supporting its effectiveness, as well as research demonstrating genetic glitches in melatonin pathways in autism.

Sensory integration methods can help with sleep.

Night terrors, though terrifying for you, are not harmful to your child, since they are not remembered in the morning (which is why many experts suggest you not mention them to your child). The most important thing you can do is keep your child safe by using gates to restrict stairs and/or doors to the outside in case they sleepwalk, and remove anything fragile or potentially dangerous from the bedroom. You might want to gently wake your child an hour after bedtime with a reassuring hug and kiss—sometimes this can disturb the child's sleep pattern enough to prevent an attack. Some parents have also found that keeping their child's feet uncovered at bedtime or even wiping cold water on their feet during an attack is enough to disrupt the event without waking the child. And remember that most children will grow out of night terrors eventually.

Seizures can also disrupt sleep, so identifying adequately and treating seizures should help with sleep.

Sleeping well is also a great stress reducer, so getting better sleep can create a positive circle of good things making more good things possible, to counteract all those vicious circles.

SEIZURES AND EPILEPSY

Seizures are an extreme case of brain overexcitation, and they're quite common in autism. Studies find seizure activity in anywhere from 7 to 46 percent of people with autism, compared to 1 to 2 percent of the general population.

Seizures happen when large groups of neurons fire together instead of in a much more varied and individualized rhythm. Once someone starts having seizures, changes occur in the brain tissue making further seizures more likely. Excitations can drive seizures, and seizures can drive excitation—each can cause more of the other. They also wreak havoc on mitochondria and cause huge amounts of oxidative stress.

It isn't always obvious when a seizure is happening. People think that seizures mean someone falls to the floor, arms flailing and eyes rolling back in their sockets. That's called a "grand mal" seizure. But there are other kinds of seizures whose signs are more subtle. Sudden spacing out and unresponsiveness might be a sign of seizure activity, as well as abrupt unprovoked aggression (though there may be other reasons for this, too).

Some kinds of seizures occur at night and interfere with normal sleep, so that even though someone may look asleep, parts of the brain are firing in lockstep coordination, with too much intensity—rather than engaging in the normal electrical rhythms of sleep. The person wakes up the next morning feeling as if they hadn't slept at all.

A much larger proportion of children with autism, even those who don't have any evidence of formal seizures, may have some abnormal electrical activity in their brains. This electrical activity is measured by an EEG test, or electroencephalogram. If too many neurons are firing at once, you can see a "spike." In some people the brain rhythms may be too slow or too fast.

In years past, neurologists were trained not to worry too much about electrical "spikes" on an EEG if they were not associated with any clear clinical problems. These days, more neurologists are wondering if we really can be sure that spikes without seizures or even the atypical rhythms are totally okay. These blips might affect brain function and information processing in ways that are subtle, but perhaps still important. Some kinds of nighttime seizures have also been considered "benign" because they go away with age. But now research is raising the possibility that even these types of seizures may impact attention, learning, emotions, or behavior.

This is another example of the "gray zone" that I've been talking about in every chapter of this book. This altered electrical activity (technically called "subclinical seizures," or changes even milder than that) is somewhere between "normal" and "disease"—a kind of "dysfunction" that may matter, depending on the person and on where you decide to draw the line about what's important.

EPILEPSY AND AUTISM HAVE A LOT IN COMMON

Autism is a syndrome with unusual behaviors that is often accompanied by epilepsy. Epilepsy is a problem with brain waves that for many people may come with learning or behavioral problems, including autism. Frances Jensen, of Children's Hospital Boston, even talks about the "epilepsy spectrum disorder" that may arise from a cascade of biological events. Is this a coincidence?

Scientists are starting to find overlap between "autism genes" and "epilepsy genes," many of which make the cells more excitable. When autism starts with regression, it often occurs between the first and second birthday, a period of time when the brain has more excitability than at any other point in life.

In addition, people with autism or epilepsy are likely to have inflammation in their brains. Seizures can be aggravated by body inflammation as well.

Inflammation triggers your immune system to send "pro-inflammatory cytokines" into the blood; these reach the brain by crossing the blood-brain barrier. This inflames the brain, making brain cells more excitable. The more excitable brain cells are, the more easily they can cross a tipping point and start to seize. Even before they cross that tipping point, they may make normal sensations become more intense, and may interfere with sleep.

Perhaps sensory, sleep, and seizure issues are all linked in a spectrum of problems with the brain's cellular excitability.

Stopping Seizures

Right now it is not standard procedure to give every child with autism an EEG, which measures brain waves, although I think things may move in that direction. I personally think it's good to get a baseline EEG. If you wonder whether your child might have some hidden seizures, or if your child regresses and loses language or other skills he or she used to have, talk with your doctor about an EEG, or a sleep EEG. Keep in mind that EEGs may miss seizures if there isn't any unusual activity during their EEG test, or if the source of the seizure is very deep in the brain. As I noted above, I also think a lot of kids with autism might be having "gray zone" brain electrical problems—too mild to meet the formal definition of seizures, but enough to interfere with their quality of life. Over time, more complex ways of analyzing these EEGs will give us better measures of the gray zone and may even predict treatments (that's part of the work we do in my TRANSCEND research program).

Remember that not every child showing a mild EEG abnormality should be on an anti-epileptic drug. Neurologists don't like to prescribe seizure drugs if they can't confirm a significant seizure disorder, because the medications can all have significant side effects. On the other hand,

---

BRAIN TESTS

EEG

An EEG measures brain waves. EEG stands for *electroencephalogram*—a picture of the brain's electricity. Electrical leads connected to wires are attached to the head. They can detect electricity from the brain. Certain rhythms are normal for waking; others are normal for sleeping. If rhythms are abnormal there may be a brain problem. Sometimes you need other kinds of brain tests to figure out what the problem may be.

MRI

MRI stands for *magnetic resonance imaging*. It takes pictures of the inside of the brain. It can help determine whether things are in the right place, whether they are the right size, whether the chemicals are in the right proportions, how the blood is flowing, and more. If an EEG shows that abnormal electrical brain waves start in one part of the brain, an MRI can be used to see if that part of the brain has any physical problems that could be causing this.

you may be able to improve things somewhat by addressing food, toxin, bugs, and stress issues.

Anti-epilepsy or anti-seizure drugs generally work by affecting how certain chemicals get in and out of brain cells. Some of these drugs deplete nutrients such as folic acid, carnitine, vitamin B_6, vitamin D, or biotin; you can ask your doctor whether your child should receive supplements to compensate for this. You should report any signs of side effects to your doctor right away. If your child is on seizure medications it is very important to be strict about staying on schedule with the doses. If an anti-seizure drug needs to be stopped it's often important to do so gradually.

There is some evidence that various nondrug approaches such as the use of vitamin B_6, magnesium, taurine, and fish oil supplements may reduce the severity or frequency of seizures. But please remember that these approaches do *not* reliably treat seizures and are *not* a substitute for solid medical treatment under the direction of your doctor. Even so, I do think that whole-body strategies—eating a healthy nutrient-dense, plant-based diet, and avoiding toxins, allergens, and infections—are a prudent baseline approach for reducing the inflammation and excitation that can lead to seizures.

Some people have found that their children's seizures become less frequent or severe or even stop after they give up gluten. A diet approach that has become standard over the past decade and a half for severe and otherwise untreatable seizures is a high-fat, low-carbohydrate "ketogenic" diet, but this diet is dangerous without extremely close medical supervision. The Modified Atkins diet is milder and may help with seizures, but also requires medical supervision. It's interesting that both of these medical diets involve drastically restricting carbs, which along the way eliminates gluten, along with increasing fat.

If you wish to try natural diet or nondrug approaches, make sure that your doctor knows exactly what you are doing, because you want to avoid doing anything that may interfere with your child's medications.

Persistent seizures that respond poorly to treatment may be a sign of another problem, such as an inborn error of metabolism (red flags for this were listed in chapter 2). If your child is having these problems you can talk to your doctor about getting a specialized workup.

When he was six, Jimmy was given a drug called depakote to control his seizures, but it gave him terrible migraines. Cindy took him off the drug after about six months, because of the migraines, and his seizures didn't return. The headaches kept coming, though, and were debilitating. When he was eight, Cindy added regular sessions with a chiropractor to Jimmy's regimen. Now he gets an occasional severe headache, but he's had only one migraine in the past year.

While chiropractors are licensed and often reimbursed by insurance, doctors and especially neurologists are often leery of them due to risks of spine and spinal cord injury and strongly discourage their patients from using this approach. Yet many parents report their child gets relief from headaches and even seizures from treatment by chiropractors, cranial osteopaths, or craniosacral-trained massage therapists. There is a small amount of literature with some sets of case histories giving modest support for these approaches. They can be very gentle and many practitioners do not use the high-velocity "adjustments" that make doctors so opposed to them.

Such treatments are aimed at releasing subtle tension in muscles, bones, and connective tissues, as well as pressure on nerves and blood vessels that could impair brain function. In that sense they are aimed at the "gray zone" of dysfunction, which is probably not an area of focus for an epilepsy specialist.

WORDS AND COMMUNICATION

Speech and Language

Speech and language problems may come from many things. The sensory overload that I described above might be one reason language is such a challenge for some kids with autism. The child may be so overwhelmed by the sounds of speech that she can't sort them out into syllables and words. The sounds may reverberate in her brain and get sorted out at very different rates than for neurotypical people. If she can make out the words, she still may be so overwhelmed by information that she can't grasp on to one idea to articulate, or one thing to respond to. Or, like Ana Todd, the noise or "static" may cut in and out, so that words come in fragments rather than continuously, making it hard to keep track of the meaning.

Speech and language problems may also come from issues with the brain's control of the mouth and tongue. Nerve signals may be weak, or poorly coordinated. Some children may have trouble with the structure of the mouth itself, such as a "tethered" tongue that can't lift properly because the membrane under it is too tight. Dental problems may also contribute to speech difficulty. Other children may have trouble coordinating their breathing and air column with their mouth, tongue, and brain.

Seizures may be another obvious or hidden cause of speech and language problems.

Sometimes children make sounds without being able to make words. I knew a patient like this whose therapist put cotton gauze on the end of a wooden tongue depressor, put it into the child's mouth, and asked him to make high-pitched vowel sounds and listen to how the sounds changed when his tongue went into different positions in his mouth. The child's face lit up as he heard different sounds coming out of his mouth when his tongue curled or flattened or touched the roof of his mouth. He started playing with his tongue as he had never done before, and in a few weeks the words that had been stuck in his head started coming out of his mouth.

Not Talking

Jimmy says that back when he was "in" autism, his brain wouldn't let him speak. He was totally nonverbal around the time of his seizures and temper tantrums. The doctor who diagnosed him with autism told Cindy that Jimmy would never be able to talk, would never improve, would never say "I love you."

But I'm not aware of scientific support for saying "never." We don't know specifically why Jimmy wasn't able to speak before. The fact that he can now shows us that the wiring was there, just obstructed somehow. His older brother had a speech delay, not learning to talk until he was four, though he had no other developmental problems. Maybe they both had similar vulnerabilities, but if so, Jimmy must have had some extra triggers that pushed him further and created other issues.

Poor Pronunciation

Not hearing words clearly or having problems using the mouth can contribute to poor pronunciation. A good speech and language assessment can help sort this out.

Not Talking but Understanding Everything

A child who can't talk may still understand your language. Your child may be picking up on more than you ever imagined. Some nonverbal children learn to use assistive communication devices or computers, and prove to have rich language abilities and to be full of fresh perceptions. One teenager with autism, named Carly Fleischmann, was nonverbal and completely locked in until she was ten and began learning some basic keyboarding skills. Her parents were astounded to realize how "with it" she really was. She was following everything; she just couldn't show how much she knew until technology helped out.

Verbal Apraxia

Carly's problem is called "verbal apraxia." In this disorder, the brain is trying to send instructions to make words, but the mouth can't carry out those instructions, probably because there is a signaling glitch along the way. As I mentioned in chapter 4, some children see some improvement in verbal apraxia when they take essential fatty acids, vitamin E, or

"DISCONNECTION" DOESN'T MEAN INTELLECTUAL DEFICIT

For years people have assumed that autism is a "disorder" based on mental "deficiency." Researchers have studied what people with autism *can't* do. Geneticists have hunted for genes associated with mental impairment to explain autism.

But a growing number of scientists are taking issue with the idea that autism is mainly about deficits and mental retardation.

Mike Merzenich, a professor of neuroscience at UC San Francisco, told the magazine *Wired* that the notion that 75 percent of autistic people are mentally retarded is "incredibly wrong and destructive." He has worked with a number of brilliant autistic children, many of whom are nonverbal and would have been plunked into the low-functioning category. "We label them as retarded because they can't express what they know," and then, as they grow older, we accept that they "can't do much beyond sit in the back of a warehouse somewhere and stuff letters in envelopes."

When people with autism do something well or even better than neurotypical individuals, it is often explained away as a consequence of another area where they are weak.

Perhaps we're dealing not with intelligence problems then, but with a communication gap. Maybe, like Carly, most people with autism are just as smart as the rest of us, but for various reasons are unable to show it in typical ways.

That's basically what a group of Canadian researchers found in 2007. Laurent Mottron, Michelle Dawson, and their colleagues tested thirty-eight children on two intelligence tests, the Wechsler Intelligence Scale and Raven's Progressive Matrices. Both are equally reputable, but the Wechsler requires greater communication skills. Children with autism averaged 30 points higher on the Raven's test than on the Wechsler scale of intelligence (some even scored 70 points higher), the scientists showed. The Wechsler suggested that 70 percent or more had cognitive deficits; the Raven showed just 20 percent in this range—meaning the vast majority of kids with autism were of normal intelligence.

both; zinc has been added for its contribution to motor planning. These substances may help by improving the nerve signals. Again, if there is improvement, it means the basic machinery is there but its use is obstructed. Many nonverbal people with autism and verbal apraxia, like Carly, have communication problems, not intelligence problems.

Losing Language

A child can experience an abrupt or gradual loss of language. If this happens it's important to get an EEG. Loss of language might be a sign that your child is developing a hidden seizure disorder. Landau-Kleffner syndrome is one such form of epilepsy where children lose language and often become autistic—but they don't necessarily have obvious seizures, so getting the EEG test is important.

Children who have regressions—who seem to be developing well and then slow down, stop developing, or even lose skills that they'd gained—are particularly likely to lose language.

Promoting Speech and Language

Because communication problems are so endemic in autism, a speech-language pathologist or **speech therapist** is often the first professional to see and suspect the condition. A speech therapist is generally the earliest or one of the earliest specialists to work with children on the spectrum, and therapy should be started as soon as possible. Therapy can help a child overcome communication problems, regardless of whether he or she can speak. In one-on-one sessions, a speech therapist will address your child's current communication needs, perhaps teaching simple sign language to young children or offering assistive technologies to older ones. A therapist might also work on pronunciation, practice conversational skills, or suggest facial exercises to help with coordination.

Since there are so many possible reasons for speech problems it's important to sort out where the problems are coming from. The first thing is to get a **hearing test.** If your child is not responding to you when you call him, it's probably related to the autism, but if it's actually due to any form of deafness you will need to pursue an additional set of therapies.

Another problem you can test for is **central auditory processing disorder** (CAPD), wherein the ear works fine but the brain has trouble processing the sound information. Treatments for this disorder may include using electronic devices to assist listening, training the child to listen more effectively by teaching him specific active listening and problem-solving skills, and/or working with a therapist.

In many cases **addressing physical or medical problems** may allow the child to resolve speech problems on his or her own. Perhaps a child's teeth are so misaligned that there's no room for the tongue. Or the muscle tone in the face is too weak to allow speech, because of mitochondrial problems. Or the brain is too full of noise or even subclinical seizures, making coherent speech impossible. In cases like this, speech therapy may be much more effective after the physical or medical problems are addressed.

If reading problems emerge later, they may have roots in earlier sensory, speech, or language problems. They may also have roots in visual problems. A child may have trouble getting the images from each eye to converge into one image, and this may slow him or her down. An assessment by a **developmental optometrist** may identify visual problems interfering with reading or learning. While many doctors consider these professionals to be controversial, they do offer a program to address use of the eyes and not just acuity of vision. For children with autism, the brain and motor system may create a lot of problems with the use of the eyes as well as other senses. Visual problems can also contribute to learning problems earlier in life.

As Jimmy said, his brain wouldn't let him speak. But he "learned" to talk within two weeks of taking milk out of his diet, Cindy says. First he spoke in single words. Then, a few months later, after they took him off gluten, Jimmy began speaking in full sentences. Certainly not every child will improve as much as Jimmy did with these dietary changes. But since dietary and nutritional changes may reduce the triggers for brain problems like inflammation (which may interfere with brain processing for speech), it doesn't surprise me to hear that Jimmy's speech improved this way.

Children who improve like this don't generally take as long to reach age-level speech than if they were learning from scratch. Maybe they've already figured language out in their brains but just needed someone to take the obstructions to speech out of the way.

Communication

Impaired communication isn't quite the same as having language issues. Someone with good language can still have problems communicating.

Echolalia—Repeating Things

Your child may sound like he or she is developing language, but it may be confined to repeating things they've heard on videos or TV. Sometimes children will repeat a phrase from a movie that contains an emotion they wish to express, rather than expressing it directly in relation to what is going on now. In one example I heard about recently, a student with autism became upset with his teacher and loudly said: "Go to hell, Lieutenant!" He had apparently been watching the movie *A Few Good Men* quite often, and this phrase was used in the same emotional context as the boy was experiencing.

Echolalia may indicate that your child is processing things in big chunks rather than breaking them down into pieces (meaningful words, meaningful tones of voice). You need finer-grained pieces to be able to move them around and use them in whatever order you choose.

If your child gets echolalic during the day, it may be a sign that he or she is getting stressed out or anxious.

Rigid Language Routines

Your child may use stock phrases even when they are not appropriate. They may always introduce themselves even to their own family members. Some children can talk at great length about their area of special interest, but not be bothered to talk about other things. Or they give monologues about their area of interest but are unable to have a back-and-forth conversation about it with another person.

Poor Nonverbal Communication

Many people with autism do not use a lot of gestures along with their speech. They may not make the facial expressions that neurotypical people expect when they talk, and the "melody" or "prosody" of their voice may seem robotic. They may not understand that tone of voice can change the meaning of things, as in the difference between a loud command and a soft request. And they may not read other people's body language. They often have a hard time picking up the signs that they are boring the person they are speaking to. Scientists from MIT have been developing technologies to help children with autism "get" these nonverbal cues. They have made glasses, for instance, that "read" the facial expressions of a conversation partner and communicate them to the wearer—showing a yellow dot or vibrating in their pocket when the other person is getting bored, and a red one when it's definitely time to change the topic. These are not yet available for purchase, but hopefully something like them will be someday.

Not "Getting" Jokes and Metaphors

A joke may depend on two different meanings of a word, on tone of voice, or on some kind of discrepancy between expectations and reality. A metaphor requires the listener to figure out what two seemingly unrelated things have in common, or to move away from literal meanings. Clichés are similarly challenging. "All the world's a stage" may be very hard to understand if you think in pictures and immediately conjure up an image of a globe and a stage with lights.

People with autism can often take these things literally and be perplexed or even angry when you talk about "throwing the baby out with the bathwater," for instance. Jokes and slang can be sources of misunderstanding between neurotypical and autistic people. Of course neurotypicals may also miss jokes that people with autism find hysterically funny. Judy Endow writes about being amused as a child by watching dust particles dancing in the light—but her neurotypical family members never "got" why she was giggling. The Groden Center in Rhode Island is now offering classes teaching humor to people with autism.

INTENSE FOCUS

We all want to be loved and appreciated for who we are. Right now, if your little boy is obsessed with elevators, then by all means go ride an elevator with him. But be sure that you **understand** what he's really excited about. There might be a hundred things about an elevator to capture your child's interest—the feeling of moving up and down, the buttons that light up when you push them, the smell of the oil lubricating the cables, the doors opening and closing. Once you figure it out, try investigating that passion more. Maybe there's a book on the history of elevators that you can share. Or a mechanical drawing that shows how one works. Or a factory in a nearby town where they make elevators. Or maybe discovering that it's the lights that are of real interest—and that they happen to have been first encountered in an elevator—will help you find other places that can delight your child in the same way.

The closer you can get to what's really inspiring your child, the more you can share the joy that he or she derives from it, and the happier you both will be. Your interest will validate his or her passion. His enthusiasm will help you be what you've always wanted to be—a "normal" parent taking pleasure in the joys and successes of your child.

Once you fully join their world and really appreciate their fascination, you can gently, slowly, and sensitively start showing your child the bridges between this intense interest and other things in the world. Reading *Charlie and the Chocolate Factory* and its sequel *Charlie and the Great Glass Elevator* with a child who loves elevators could open up entirely new worlds, as the elevator bursts through the factory roof and up into the sky. It might spur an interest in space exploration or bird's-eye views, and then satellites. If you do this delicately, your son or daughter will start to feel safe enough to expand his or her interests and connections to the world on their own.

STRESS

Stress Propels Vicious Circles

As we already learned from Ana Todd, language problems can create their own stress. Ana was so worried about saying something stupid, inappropriate, or mangled that she often kept her mouth shut.

The anxiety also carried over into the rest of her life—she lived in a state of constant worry. That stress, as I'm sure you've guessed by now, likely fed on itself and created even more problems for her.

Every nervous system issue I've told you about in this chapter may contribute to stress. Too much sensory stimulation, trouble being coordinated, not enough sleep, seizures, not being able to say what you want—all can contribute to frustration and stress. Looking for solutions at each of these levels can help reduce the stress and increase the time spent truly learning and enjoying life.

The brain is an astonishing "computer" that thinks and feels, and it is a physical organ that can be healthy or sick. It generates behaviors and processes information. It also generates seizures, sleep problems, sensory disorders, hormone problems, stress, oxidative stress, and inflammation.

A whole-body, intense-world view of autism shows you how interconnected things are:

- Speech problems are mysteriously made better during bouts of fever;
- More sleep can lead to fewer tantrums and seizures and less sensory overload;
- Getting seizures under control can improve sleep and sensory processing;
- And many of these problems seem to get milder with measures to improve cellular health.

Depending on how complicated or severe your child's brain problems are, the measures I am suggesting in this book may not be enough to calm the chaos.

But it's not an all-or-nothing thing.

Every bit of relief you give to this highly stressed and overwhelmed system could give some part of it a chance to do better than it did before. Whole-body strategies are aimed at reducing risk as much as possible so your child's potential for health and well-being has the best chance to shine through.

In the next chapter I will tell you about how to take your new insights into whole-body and brain features of autism and use them to connect with your child and understand and transform their behaviors.

KEEP IN MIND

- Brain problems are a really big deal.
- Addressing and reducing brain problems can help both behavior and health.
- It's important to get appropriate medical attention for brain problems.
- You can also help reduce some of the things that worsen brain problems by helping with whole-body problems.
- Brain differences are not always brain problems.

But also remember

- Brain problems are not the only problems in autism.
- There is hope for improvements even if you don't totally fix all the brain problems.
- All brains do *not* have to be normal in the same way.
- Even if symptoms of autism largely go away, a person's perceptions and insights may still be distinctive, which can be a source of talent and provide valuable contributions to the world.

PART III

Transcend Autism: Share the Strengths and Lose the Pain

CHAPTER 7

Join Your Child's World

S ometimes, when sitting in a chair, Judy Endow loses her body. She worries she'll topple over, because she can't feel herself in space.

Recently she was invited into a fourth-grade classroom to observe a boy who was being disruptive. While Judy and several school officials watched, the boy started tapping his foot loudly.

The teacher very nicely asked him to stop and explained that the class needed quiet time right now for reading.

A few seconds later, the boy popped out of his seat and ran around the room. When chased down, he started giggling and pulling away.

By this time his classmates were completely distracted, and the teacher was beside herself. The teacher again explained to the boy in front of the whole class why his behavior was inappropriate.

Judy, an educational consultant who has autism herself, tried a different approach. She gently took the boy's hands and asked him to jump with her. After jumping for a little while she asked him if he'd had enough or wanted to jump more. "More," he said. So they did. Then she asked him again, and again he wanted more. After a few minutes he was ready to stop jumping, sit quietly in his seat, and read productively for the remainder of the reading session.

Judy advised this teacher that it would be easier to make progress with the boy if she stopped thinking about how his behavior was "bad" and instead tried to imagine what needs he was trying to meet by behaving this way.

This was the question Judy had asked herself when the boy was running around the room. Because of her professional training and her own sensory experiences, Judy is better than most neurotypical people are at figuring out the needs of kids with autism. She guessed that this boy had probably lost the sense of what it feels like to have a body and was worried he'd fall out of his chair. He started tapping his foot and then running around so that, through movement, he could reclaim his physical sensations. By jumping with him, Judy helped him regain those feelings, and then he could learn again.

"When I look at someone and they are behaving strangely, what I do is I [think] 'If I were doing that, it would be because of this, this, or this,'" Judy said. "So in a very simplistic way I can guess why they are doing what they are doing."

Meeting Your Child Where She Lives

I think Judy's work is a terrific example of how meeting a child where he or she is can make a tremendous difference. By understanding why your child is acting this way instead of blaming them for acting in a way you wouldn't, you can start to approach them with curiosity rather than judgment. I'd rather spend time with someone who is interested in me than with someone who is trying to fix me or always telling me to do stuff that doesn't make sense. Wouldn't you?

In this chapter I want to help you see, as Judy does, that your child's behavior is not "bad," irrational, or meant to upset you. Instead it is behavior that has some meaning or some purpose to your child, no matter how odd or irrational it may seem to you. Once you figure out that logic, you will be able to help your child much more effectively, while also dramatically reducing your own frustration.

Judy was able to guess correctly because her nervous system issues are similar to the boy's. However, as a neurotypical person, you will have a harder time making accurate guesses, because the experience of living in your body is probably very different from his; if you were doing that behavior it would likely be for a very different reason. Understanding how your child's brain is overactivated and hypersensitive can help you bridge from what your own body is telling you to what your child's body is telling him or her. You will probably guess best about the meaning of your child's behavior when you look at what he or she is doing from the point of view of a person with an inconsistent sensory system.

As much as your child needs stability and order, your life is regularly and unpredictably upended by the latest crisis. He might suddenly become interested in feeling that stuff that comes exploding out of his backside, and you discover him—and the bathroom—smeared in feces. She might throw a temper tantrum the day you really needed her out of the house, and be so exhausted that she has to stay home, wrapped in your arms. Your other children might rebel in some choice way to the attention you necessarily lavish on your "needier" kid.

I'd like to talk about ways to minimize those parental moments of sheer horror and terror and maximize the ones that remind you why you wanted to become a parent in the first place.

It may seem unfair that this burden falls on you. Why can't your kid figure out the world the way everyone else's does? You're right. It's not fair. But don't take that unfairness out on your child by getting frustrated or angry at how slowly he learns the ways of the world. Instead help him do it better and more richly—more sensitively—and don't worry about the speed; that will come by itself later. You can help him best by trying to see that world as he does and using that insight to help you translate your world to him.

There's been a lot of research about how people with autism lack a so-called theory of mind—they don't understand that you are a different person with different needs than theirs. That may be true, but teachers, parents, and specialists are often just as lacking in their understanding of what might be called the child's theory of sensation and perception. You don't "get" why she experiences a flickering lightbulb as a bolt of lightning, a doorbell ringing as the sound of a thousand church bells. You don't appreciate why a child might need to tap his foot and run around the classroom to keep from falling out of his chair. And you don't grasp how yogurt, because of its smoothness, may be one of the only foods that doesn't make your daughter feel like she has a mouthful of pebbles.

Your child may have as hard a time figuring out your needs as you have figuring out hers. She may not notice that today is a bad day for

Judy finds it disturbing that her view of the world is seen as "wrong," while the neurotypical view is always right. Here's what she once told me via email:

"Sometimes I get frustrated because it seems all the onus is on *me* learning the neurotypical ways of thinking and then matching myself to their ways of thinking in order to be in step with them. And then, even though I am the one doing all the work to learn *their* theory of mind and then try to match them, they often blame me for not having their theory of mind.

"I think it would be nice if neurotypicals could understand that I do have my own theory of mind. How I think and respond to situations, though different from how they think and respond, does not make me less than a human being. It just makes me different.

"When autistics are judged by the measure of neurotypical theory of mind, they come up short. If the people of the world were judged according to my theory of mind they would all measure up deficient. Because there are fewer autistics than neurotypicals, we have to live with their perceptions and theory of mind as the standard, which in turn makes us deviant.

"Maybe it would be more helpful to learn each other's theories of mind rather than only having neurotypicals try to drum into autistics their theory of mind as if they have the correct standard."

you, and so try to be less needy. He may talk endlessly because he can't read your cues of boredom.

Search for the Hidden Meaning

So, once again, it's time to put on your sleuthing hat and become a detective. Now, many of your child's behaviors may not make obvious sense—they don't seem to serve any clear purpose. But your child doesn't smear poop all over the walls "on purpose" to make you cry or get angry. Assume for a minute that "crazy" behaviors like this do make some sense, that your child is sending you coded messages about things that are important to him—and your job is to break the code so you can "read" the messages.

By paying attention differently to these actions, you may be able to notice clues you didn't see before, and find a more effective way to help your child. Taking this approach will also help you respond more carefully to these "bizarre" behaviors, so you don't inadvertently reinforce them by rewarding your child for activities that drive you up the wall.

The first thing to do is to start recording these outbursts and stunts the way an anthropologist might record the actions of a newly discovered native people. Suspend your judgments, what you think you know. What time do these events most often happen? Does the same thing often happen first? Perhaps he's more likely to have outbursts on pizza day in the school cafeteria, or after you've just turned on the lights because it's getting dark outside. Maybe it only happens when you turn on the fluorescent light in the kitchen. Many behaviors are set off or triggered by an event. Just as you might suddenly feel hungry as you walk past a bakery, there are "setting events" in your child's life—the things that "set off" difficult behaviors. You can use a diary or log to try to identify these setting events for some of your child's most difficult behaviors.

One mother I know noticed, after hunting for setting events, that her son was having more temper tantrums in the afternoon. He never told her he was hungry, but after she started giving him a snack when she picked him up at school, the outbursts largely disappeared.

Think of Jimmy from chapter 6, who would pitch a fit when he approached a restaurant with a flickering neon sign. His mother later realized that Jimmy wasn't against going out to eat, but that the sign was triggering a seizure. Again, instead of random acts of seeming insanity, these outbursts are your child's way of telling you something about the external environment—the sights, sounds, smells, and sensory stimuli around him—or his internal environment—for example, allergies, stomach pains, or seizure activity.

The late Dr. Edward G. Carr of Stony Brook University in New York spent his career researching the communication role of these seemingly bizarre and/or self-destructive behaviors. A psychologist, Carr helped develop two strategies for dealing with autism—"Functional Behavior Assessment" and "Positive Behavior Support"—that are now recommended by the federal government. His core message was *"fix contexts,* not *behaviors*." Instead of looking at the behavior as "bad," look for how the context, or environment, is out of synch with your child, and explore what you can do about it.

External Environment

Some things in your child's surroundings are changeable and some are not.

Sometimes the problem is a well-meant gesture that's actually counterproductive, like a teacher popping a candy in your daughter's mouth to keep her quiet, unintentionally rewarding her for being loud in class.

Sometimes just figuring out what the problem is can help you do something about it. Your refrigerator will always make humming noises, but if you realize that sound is distracting your hearing-sensitive son, you can help him set up a quieter spot to do homework.

Sometimes you will find a mismatch between what's expected of your child and what she can actually do. In her wonderful memoir, *Strange Son,* Portia Iversen recalls her realization that her nonverbal son knew how to read—in both English and Hebrew—even though his teachers thought he still didn't know his letters. Once Iversen realized this disconnect and matched her son's education to his needs, he acted out much less.

Sensory stimulation: Your child may respond with disruptive behavior if he's being overwhelmed by too much sensory information. Jimmy from chapter 6 is a bright boy with a lot of energy for learning. But he has a classmate who cries for hours each day. The sound and the emotional weight of that crying pushes Jimmy over the edge and makes it very difficult for him to concentrate and learn. His mother has realized this and is trying to switch him into a classroom that will be less disruptive.

Social triggers: Maybe your daughter realizes she has no friends, so recess time is particularly tough for her. Talking to the teacher and even her classmates might make a difference. Tell them what your daughter's problems are and enlist their help. Yes, kids can be cruel to one another but they can also be phenomenally open and accepting. Reach out to their better natures. Don't assume they should know how to behave around your child, but teach them how and you may be astounded by how supportive her peers become.

Communication problems: Maybe your son is frustrated because he can't communicate—about either the bad reflux that's hurting his throat, or the question he'd like to answer on the blackboard. Using pictures, sign language, or a keyboard instead of talking might help. Here's where experimentation and a great teacher can make all the difference.

Interests: Maybe your child tunes out because the teacher or the material isn't engaging. If your son's preschool class is spending the year talking about dinosaurs and he's obsessed with machines, maybe the teacher can steer the topic a bit in his direction, spending some class time talking about the machines used to study dinosaurs or dig up their bones.

Internal Environment

Dr. Carr and I wrote a paper together in 2008 about the power of integrating the biological and behavioral approaches to treatment. (Sadly, he was killed by a drunk driver the following year.) As we argued in that article, addressing just the behaviors won't help if they are caused by a physical problem. If you notice, for instance, that your teenager's aggressive behavior is linked to eating certain foods, you might wonder whether something about those foods is setting him off. It could be the foods themselves, or his diet triggering reflux, and the pain from that is spurring on his aggressive behavior. If your throat was incredibly painful because of acid reflux and you couldn't tell anyone about it (in part because your throat hurt too much), you might start banging your head against the wall, too.

If you are only thinking about behavior, and if you assume that behavior is always psychologically motivated, it won't occur to you that head banging, as well as biting and excessive scratching, are often things people with autism do when they have pain. Before you add a behavior modification program to treat the head banging, add a treatment for reflux. And remember, even when he's medicated for reflux and/or has changed his diet to avoid food that contributes to it, he may still get into problem foods or need his medication adjusted—or even have the occasional plain old bad day. And you can put off a challenging task for another day, just as you do on your own bad days.

I was monitoring an autism support chat room on the Internet recently when I came across this story, which I think makes my point beautifully:

A mother wrote about the day she picked her daughter up at the end of an occupational therapy session and the therapist wanted to talk about the girl's new "stimming" behavior. The girl had started biting her tongue repeatedly and the therapist offered to come up with a behavior modification plan to address it. Instead the mom put herself in her daughter's world and tried to understand in what context the tongue biting would make sense. She then stuck her fingers in her daughter's mouth and discovered a piece of lettuce wedged between the girl's teeth and gums. The mom removed it and the daughter's repetitive behavior was "cured."

Here are some of the places to look for clues when hunting for internal triggers of behavior problems:

Sources of pain: Look aggressively for all possible sources of pain, such as teeth, reflux, gut, broken bones, cuts and splinters, infections, abscesses, sprains, and bruises. Any behaviors that seem to be localized might indicate pain. If he always likes to sit curled up in a ball, for instance, or drapes his belly over the arm of the couch, that might be because his stomach is hurting. Ana Todd from chapter 3 thinks that her childhood obsession with lying on her stomach had something to do with gut problems that no one realized she had.

Distinguishing sensations: Remember, your child may not be able to tell you that he or she is in pain. This might be because of communication difficulties. Or it might be because they can't specifically identify the source themselves, just as Crystal from chapter 4 didn't even have the self-awareness to know when she had to poop. Maybe she's hungry or thirsty, but can't express it. This can even happen to people who appear to be functioning at a very high level.

Seizures: Some behaviors, especially those that seem particularly odd, unmotivated, abrupt, or out of nowhere, may be due to seizures. If you are concerned about this, keep a very careful record of what you observe, see if your child's teachers and therapists have similar observations, and discuss it with your doctor.

Food allergies and sensitivities: Try to identify any food allergies or sensitivities that might be bothering your child. Diarrhea within a few hours of eating a particular food could certainly indicate an allergy; so can red, flushed cheeks or ears. Many people report that their child's flapping or repetitive behaviors go away when they cut out certain foods. An elimination diet can show you for certain whether specific foods trigger pain or unusual behaviors. Whatever you do to treat gut problems could make a huge difference in your child's behavior. If your therapist uses problem foods like candies or wheat crackers as rewards during behavior therapy, your child's negative reactions to the food could outweigh their positive reactions to the therapy.

Fatigue, hunger, or thirst: As with anyone, being hungry, tired, or thirsty can make your child cranky. Poor sleep or coming down with a cold could easily explain unusual behavior. A chronic illness or low-grade infection could make her irritable. If your child has a pattern of crankiness at a certain time of day, try offering a piece of fruit at that hour to see if it makes a difference.

Emotions: Sorrow, anger, fear, and anxiety can also have an impact on behavior. Parents who are going through a divorce, a health crisis, a job change, or a move might think they're handling everything and there's no reason for their child to be concerned. But if you're stressed about something, chances are your child will be, too—particularly if he's powerless to do anything about it, or even communicate his concerns. The birth of a new child might also create emotions as well as competition for attention. Even highly verbal children often struggle to identify and interpret their emotions, and might act out sideways; "My ski boots are killing my feet" can be code for "I have no idea where my body is in space and I'm terrified I'm going to fall off the mountain." Or "This book is stupid" can mean "My anxiety makes it impossible for me to read a book about a child whose parents are dead."

Coordination problems can contribute to stress and behavior issues. As anyone who's ever been picked last or near last for a team knows, grade school gym class can be stressful. If your child has trouble undoing buttons or zippers, the short time allotted for locker room changes or bathroom breaks can add tremendous stress. When you walk awkwardly, negotiating a crowded hallway between classes can be stressful.

Many people with autism also have problems that we often associate with attention deficit/hyperactivity disorder. Overloading your child with stimuli, stress, or demands may make it even harder for her to concentrate. Pain or discomfort can also be a distraction, as can metabolic problems, gut bugs, and a poor diet.

As I hope you can appreciate by now, there are many things you can do once you look for ways to fix the context and not just the behaviors.

THE ZIGGURAT MODEL AND COMPREHENSIVE AUTISM PLANNING SYSTEM (CAPS)

The Ziggurat Model is an approach to formulating comprehensive intervention plans that addresses all the levels of needs and strengths of an individual child. Federal law mandates multidisciplinary assessment of each child, and the Ziggurat Model, which is now mandated in a number of U.S. states, as well as provinces in Canada, meets this requirement.

This model was developed in response to educators' concerns that the choice of interventions felt haphazard, and the observation that critical needs of children were often not being met.

Its five-tiered pyramid model serves as a kind of checklist to make sure all of these bases are covered.

INTERVENTION ZIGGURAT

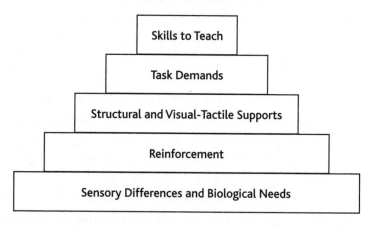

The specific interventions are designed in relation to a careful analysis of each child's individual strengths and skills and underlying characteristics. The Comprehensive Autism Planning System (CAPS) helps teams to put the model into practice in the classroom.

I work closely with a number of users of Ziggurat and CAPS models who welcome a whole-body approach to autism because it greatly fleshes out what can be done at the base of the pyramid to address Sensory Difference and Biological Needs.

Stabilization, Regulation, and Sensory Breaks

Once you have addressed your child's physical needs, it's time to consider sensory and emotional regulation. As you saw in the last chapter, your child's sensory experiences are probably very different from your own. She is likely easily overwhelmed by information coming in through some senses, perhaps upset by loud noises, and isn't getting enough input from the senses responsible for self-awareness and regulation. In school you learned about five senses: taste, smell, sound, sight, and touch. Two more senses are important to understand your child: the vestibular sense, which controls balance, and proprioception, or the sense of one's body in space. In many people with autism, some of the information from these senses is too much, too little, or distorted, leading to feelings of terror, pain, or disengagement.

To overcome the confusion, your child needs help stabilizing his senses. Occupational therapists talk about sensory diet, opportunities for sensory input that help free up the ability to do other kinds of activities. Judy Endow recommends sensory breaks—moments during the day when your child can fill sensory needs. For the boy at the beginning of the chapter, jumping up and down was a sensory break that allowed him to focus again in class. As a teenager, Temple Grandin, an animal welfare expert, author, advocate, and person with autism, built what she called a squeeze machine to help her regulate her senses. By lying in the machine and turning it on, Grandin could put pressure on most of her body at once. The steady pressure helped her feel calm, and in her body in a way that her neurology did not do on its own.

Observe your child and see what they gravitate to when they do repetitive behaviors. That might give you some clues to what sensory activities help them regroup. Depending on your child's needs and strengths, a sensory break might include: spinning, rocking, doing push-ups against the wall, rubbing something with texture, wearing a weighted vest or blanket, listening to music, sucking through a straw, chewing something crunchy, taking a visual break in a quiet environment, or using an assistive technology.

Exercise is also a great way to calm the nervous system and to teach physical self-control. Team sports that require advanced skill and social interactions probably aren't a good idea, but depending on your child's age, skills, and fears, going to the gym or the pool, rolling a ball across the floor, or heading out for a family walk or run can help reduce stress and feed sensory needs.

According to one study, the benefit of proprioceptive information lasts for about two hours, so your child might need a sensory break like this approximately every two hours. Some children need to get stabilized much more frequently. Of course every child is different and their needs are likely to change daily. Judy talks about her need to get sensory information proactively—before there's a problem—and reactively, if there's something in the moment that's causing her stress.

She wrote a book called *Practical Solutions for Stabilizing Students with Classic Autism to Be Ready to Learn: Getting to Go!,* whose title describes what it takes to prepare someone to deal with the world. Judy writes: "A person with classic autism never knows ahead of time how his nervous system will interpret incoming information or how his brain will process it. This means that the person constantly needs to be 'on guard' in terms of watching his behavioral responses—the more dysregulated they become, the more of a challenge it is to deal with even the most ordinary events of the day." The person's comfort level in everyday life, she continues, depends on how well regulated she can be that day. When she is not well regulated, her behavior will suffer. Every day she needs to pay attention to keeping herself regulated, just like we all need to brush our teeth.

One goal of therapy is for your child to develop enough self-awareness to know when they need to stabilize, self-regulate, and take a sensory break—and to know how to do these things. Then, regardless of their issues, they will manage better in the world.

AVOIDING EXPLOSIONS

Judy Endow developed these strategies when her teenage son with autism "flunked out" of a psychiatric hospital because he was having so many meltdowns.

She describes the meltdown process as a train with four cars: Starting Out, Picking Up Steam, Point of No Return, and Explosion. If they all hook up, watch out! She came up with the following strategies to avoid hookups:

1. Treat sensory problems proactively. Endow compares an autistic person's need for sensory integration activities with a diabetic's need for insulin. Unfortunately there's no autistic equivalent for a glucose monitor. Instead, she says, everyone on the spectrum who needs it should get a daily dose of sensory activities. Now in her fifties, Judy continues to do so.

2. Because autistic people tend to "think in pictures," as Temple Grandin put it, they generally benefit more from visual information than from being told to do something—particularly when they're under stress. For a child with communication problems, having a picture of a bathroom to point to may help avoid problems when he really has to go. There are many places to purchase pictures and a board to stick them on, or you can make your own.

3. Manage emotions before they get out of control. Endow says that when her sensory system is well regulated, she is less likely to magnify small emotions entirely out of proportion to reality. If she is not well regulated, she feels the same emotional intensity when her grocery store is out of her favorite food as she did when she heard about the 9/11 tragedy—even though intellectually she understands the vast gulf between the two. Self-regulation, stabilization, and sensory breaks have helped her over time to be able to rein in such "irrational" emotions. She believes others can learn to manage their emotions as well. Systematic instruction and visual supports like Kari Dunn Buron's 5-Point Scale (www.5pointscale.com, and see page 178) can also help.

Getting to Learning

It's really a basic part of human nature to be curious and to want to learn and do well. This is true of people with autism, too, of course. It's just that their nervous systems put a lot of obstacles in the way.

As you make progress in addressing your child's physical needs, resolving as much pain and removing as much environmental stress as possible, they will start having more bandwidth for learning.

Learning becomes easier when your child can see differences and patterns in their environment. This is hard to do when everything is chaos, when sensation is overwhelming. Judy talks about how all sensory information comes to her equally: The road signs and the leaves on the trees arrive to her eyes with the same level of importance, which is not very helpful when she's driving. But she has learned how to focus her attention on the salient information—the other cars and the road signs. It takes her more energy and effort than for a neurotypical person, but she can do it, and many other adults with autism talk about learning to do the same.

Education makes the world more orderly and structured. It reduces stress and increases competency.

Children with autism do not spontaneously learn many of the things that are helpful in navigating the world. They need to be taught things that are totally obvious to neurotypical people. Think about how many skills it takes simply to know how to handle yourself in a public bathroom, or to ride in an elevator—face the front, don't touch anyone, stay near the sides if there's room, push the button, flush the toilet, wash hands, acknowledge other people, but not too much . . . According to educator Brenda Smith Myles, there is a "hidden curriculum" for understanding unstated rules in social situations, and this needs to be explicitly taught to people with autism.

Some public school systems use Discrete Trial teaching or training, a form of applied behavioral analysis. This approach breaks down skills into the smallest possible tasks, which are taught one at a time. Each tiny component of the task is taught with as many repetitions as the child needs to really get it. The teacher poses a question or gives a stimulus or prompt. The child responds. The desired response is rewarded. Each repetition is a discrete trial and performance is carefully tracked and analyzed. When the child clearly can produce the desired response, the teacher can move on to the next skill. Over time the child progresses to more complex material.

However, there is still a lot of variability, not only among states and school districts, but even among teachers in the same school. You will need to be informed and alert. A good source of information on autism intervention approaches is the Autism Internet Modules, found at the OCALI (Ohio Center for Autism and Low Incidence) website, www.autisminternetmodules.org.

Skills that can be taught range broadly, and include making eye contact, shaking hands, going to the store, academics, and everything in between.

BEHAVIORAL APPROACHES FOR PICKY EATERS

I have been advising you to change the foods your child eats. How do you do this if your child is a picky eater or compulsively craves foods that are not healthy? A systematic behavioral approach can make a decisive difference.

Food issues can come from sensory reactions such as finding food smells overwhelming or textures unbearable. They can come from pain from medical conditions such as inflammation in the esophagus. The child may have a hard time using his or her mouth, teeth, and tongue in a coordinated way. Past bad experiences with food may have caused a persistent food anxiety. Unpredictability at mealtimes may make anxiety worse, as may noise and distraction, such as TV, music, or loud talking. Many children may have a lot more than one of these symptoms.

At the same time, the bad food habits may be part of what is making the child rigid, poorly coordinated, or beset by sensory issues.

Your challenge is to solve this by getting your child to change from bad to good food habits. What does it take for your autistic child to accept new foods?

Take a tip from the Discrete Trial approach and *break the process down into tiny steps, offering tiny rewards for each successfully completed step.*

Start with what *is* working about eating, no matter how small—like catching a kid being good—and start from there with positive reinforcement. Once the child knows what it is that adults are after they tend to do more of it.

To introduce a new food:

- Choose the food.
- Involve your child in picking a reinforcer—also known to parents everywhere as a "bribe." This should be an inducement appropriate to the task. Don't promise a hundred-dollar present with every new food tried unless you're willing to donate the family fortune very quickly. Make sure it's something of interest to your child, such as a sticker of a beloved kind of animal, or a bit of their favorite food. And allow your child to help choose the reinforcer when possible—perhaps among a few options you present.

- Approach your child gently and slowly. First show the food. Gradually advance to putting it in your child's hand. Touch it to your child's lips. Don't try to go straight for accepting the food, chewing, and swallowing it—that's like going from zero to 100 mph in ten seconds.
- At first reinforce the child not only for eating the bite of food, but also for behaviors that involve exploring it, such as touching it with hands, taking it in the mouth, and spitting it out.
- Reinforce the responses you want, such as tasting the new food, but remember, don't reinforce or react to the responses you don't want, such as throwing it against the wall.
- If a specific trial fails, don't get mad. Keep things calm. Proceed to the next trial.
- Keep data. Take each trial as a unit and track what happens.
- Be persistent over long periods of time. All children need to be presented with new foods as much as a dozen or more times, and a child with autism may need even more reinforcement to turn a new food into a favorite. If you persist you will get solid results.
- If the situation becomes truly dire, there are feeding programs run by professionals.

Intensive Behavioral Intervention

Applied behavioral analysis (ABA) is the only behavioral treatment in autism that is well supported by data so far, and it can be a valuable tool for adding structure, predictability, and skills to your child's life. It is often available as part of the services your child may be entitled to in your state, depending on the laws and regulations; however, there are often shortages of qualified therapists and programs.

Recently other approaches have been researched and data is emerging. Pivotal response therapy, for example, is a variant of ABA that targets critical areas of a child's development and functioning, such as motivation, being able to respond to social cues, and initiating social interaction. By targeting these "pivotal" competencies this approach aims to create impacts in domains beyond what is specifically targeted, and there are some studies to support that it can do this.

Research suggests that nearly every child can benefit from behavioral therapy. Please remember that biological therapies are not a substitute for behavioral therapies. Both are usually necessary to treat the whole child.

Some therapies won't work, however, if your child isn't ready for them, as Caleb wasn't when his mother, Joy, tried a variation called Floortime with him from ages two to four. Floortime is about playing with a child on the floor in his space to build a relationship. But Caleb wasn't yet ready to relate to someone else, because his sense of his own body was so confused and he couldn't pay attention. Later, when he was more connected to his body and had had a lot of ABA, he was able to make much more progress in building relationships.

The point is that the method you choose needs to be appropriate to where your child is now. A child isn't ready to learn social skills when he can't feel his own body. A child can't focus when she is distracted by a stomachache. A child won't sit still in class if sensory needs are driving him wild.

This also means that your child may outgrow or max out on a therapy and you will need to transition to some new approaches.

AVOIDING BEHAVIOR PROBLEMS

Here are a dozen commonsense tips from Brenda Smith Myles, a prominent applied autism researcher and educator, for doing an end run around behavior problems:

1. Don't rush. You need to operate on autism time rather than expecting your child to act on yours.
2. Take more time to do fewer things. A rough rule of thumb is that people with autism take twice the time to accomplish half as much.
3. Provide structure and spell out routines through pictures, stories, or other reinforcement.
4. Take frequent breaks. Leave time for relaxation.
5. Anticipate physical needs, such as bathroom and eating breaks, and provide for them ahead of time.

6. Have a clear plan and routine, but be ready to change it and help the child with the change. Offer structured predictability.
7. Teach calming skills.
8. Respect your child's interests and abilities and give them space.
9. Praise your child abundantly.
10. "Live out loud"—narrate what you are doing and why you are doing it, and problem-solve out loud, too.
11. Use daily activities and events to teach basic information that your child may not learn spontaneously.
12. Don't forget to laugh! Having fun with your child is the best revenge you can take against whatever got you in this position in the first place.

THE 5-POINT SCALE

The Incredible 5-Point Scale, developed by Kari Dunn Buron, teaches social and emotional concepts through the use of a simple visual, making it particularly effective with nonverbal students. The scale gives the child a system for rating what's going on for them, what it feels like inside, and what they can try to do or whom they can ask for help.

Reducing Stress

There's plenty of research now confirming that people with autism suffer more from stress and anxiety than neurotypicals do. This added stress could come from some biological aspect of autism, from the confusion of not being able to understand their world, or from their awareness of and frustration with differences. Remember how much Ana Todd's awkward pattern of speech stressed her out.

What is clear is that stressful events can increase negative behaviors such as aggression, self-injury, tantrums, and repetitive behaviors, and can interfere with learning and being open to new experience.

Anxiety, of course, is another one of our vicious circles. If your daughter knows she might fall and call attention to herself when walking down the hallway at school, she might become fearful of that walk. That anxiety then makes it harder for her to walk well down the hall—and more likely to fall! Being anxious can also limit anyone's ability to pay attention, process, and learn, thereby exacerbating problems. The anxious look on a teacher's face might stress out your son, making it harder for him to focus and more likely that he'll tune out the lesson. Once he falls behind the rest of the class, that becomes its own stress.

People with autism also often lack the reserves of neurotypicals. They'll get overwhelmed and run-down faster, and they'll have a harder time calming themselves when they do get upset.

Traditionally it's been very hard to study stress in people with autism. The electrodes and MRI machines that are used to measure stress can be intolerable for test subjects. Researchers Rosalind Picard and Matthew Goodwin at the MIT Media Lab have figured out a way around this problem by developing high-tech sensors that can be worn like clothing, measuring heart rate, breathing rate, and something called electrodermal activity, which is what makes your palms sweat when you're nervous. This research has led to one stunning finding: We are often wrong about when we think an autistic person is calm or stressed out.

Goodwin, who also works at the Groden Center, a treatment and research center in Rhode Island, had used earlier technologies to discover that oftentimes when a teacher perceived a student to be perfectly calm, the student's heart rate was spiking and sweat glands were pumping, indicating high levels of stress. Goodwin and his team thought that if a simple wearable monitor were able to alert teachers to stress and anxiety that they would not have suspected, the teachers would have a better chance of preventing crises before they happened. These high-tech mini-sensors may soon be available to the general public, and more mini-devices may find their way onto the market in the next few years.

Calming Down

With her research and clinical colleagues, June Groden, cofounder of the Groden Center, has developed calming strategies and a relaxation program tailored to people with developmental disabilities. Limiting sources of stress is obviously ideal, but not always realistic. Generally relaxation techniques include a combination of breathing, imagery, and deep muscle relaxation. The Groden experts recommend learning these techniques in a nonstressful situation and then slowly teaching the person to use the skills when stressed. Using the techniques before going into a situation that will probably be stressful can also help.

In addition to being more vulnerable to stress than neurotypicals, people with autism are also stressed out by different things. They're less able to handle criticism, for instance, explains Groden, who created the center with her husband, Gerald, in 1976. And for many, the word *no* is enough to launch a tantrum.

The Groden Center teaches parents and people with autism to identify triggers and setting events. Such a "functional analysis of behavior" can be extremely helpful, Groden says, but is often done poorly at local institutions, leading teachers and parents to aim for the wrong targets.

Groden's latest book and work is about using positive psychology to reduce stress.

Groden also believes that building character and values in people with autism can help reduce stress. By teaching them to say thank you, hold doors, and help out in whatever way they can, people with autism will be able to feel better about themselves. Plus, she says, "if you're teaching a person kindness, they're going to be more accepted in the community."

Social interactions can be a huge source of stress for people with autism, and reducing that stress can be transformative. Just as you need to help your child learn to read, write, and do math problems, you also need to help his or her social skills. For younger kids, it's how to play with others on the playground; for older teens, it's how to act in a job interview. Early intervention is critical because once they fall behind, it becomes harder to catch up.

Playing Gorilla

Like most parents of kids on the spectrum, Joy from chapter 1 went through a long list of treatments and programs to try to help Caleb. Though we can't know for sure what helped in ways we can't see, one

June Groden starts helping someone with autism relax by working on big movements and muscle groups:

- First, tighten one arm, hold it, and then relax it. Do the same thing for the other arm and then for each leg.
- Then, concentrate on tightening and relaxing each hand. Many people with autism have repetitive behaviors related to their hands. When they understand how to relax their hands, they can intentionally relax them instead of flapping or flicking. Perhaps this also helps them to feel their hands better.
- Then, do some deep breathing: Inhale deeply, hold it, and then let the air out. When you get comfortable with that, add a short pause before inhaling again.
- Choose a meaningful calming word, such as *peace* or *relax,* to think about with each exhale. Practice this regularly when things are peaceful. The word then becomes associated with a relaxed feeling and can be used later to re-create that feeling even in situations of stress. Many children learn to do this on their own initiative when they notice they are getting stressed.

June Endow says she once had a very bad reaction to a yoga relaxation exercise, with her muscles getting locked in a clenched and awkward position. A bad experience like this might mean a particular technique is wrong for you, or it might mean there's something else in the way. In this case, muscle cramps might have come from a magnesium deficiency. Supplementing with magnesium might remove the obstacle. Clearly, not all strategies will work for everyone, but sometimes a simple change will make a difference.

program clearly made a profound difference for Caleb: the Son-Rise Program at the Autism Treatment Center of America, in western Massachusetts. Caleb, then eight, responded not only because of the program's strengths, but also because he was ready for what it had to offer.

The fall before starting the program Joy had cleared Caleb's diet of preservatives and allergens, getting rid of wheat, dairy, soy, egg, and corn, and having him eat mostly raw, organic foods. Whatever physical problems were caused by eating those foods had been resolved. She had also done years of work on his sensory regulation, including sensory integration therapy and auditory training to reduce his sensitivity to sounds. He was taking medication to control his anxiety. He was feeling better, but he was still lost.

"Pray for me, Mom, I don't know where I am," Caleb once told her.

Joy, a nurse, was able to work enough overtime to pay for the first installment of her training in the Son-Rise Program. She didn't know how she would possibly afford the next two sessions, but she decided to trust that if it was the right thing, God would provide it.

When she came home from the first leg of the training, she turned a room in the family's basement into Caleb's workroom. It had no distractions, just bare walls and simple carpeting.

Joy vividly remembers one day soon after setting up the room. She and Caleb were in the room, and Caleb started pounding on his chest. Instead of asking why he was pounding on his chest or trying to get him to stop, Joy, primed by the training, started pounding on hers, too.

"Within two minutes, which never happened before, he looked me straight in the eye," Joy said. She responded by praising Caleb lavishly, as she had been taught. "Thank you so much for looking at me! Let's be gorillas [together]!" They kept on playing gorilla for twenty minutes— the first time Caleb had played a game—and kept it up eons longer than he'd ever been able to focus on one activity before.

"After twenty minutes, he was done and I was totally okay with that," Joy says. She had decided to accept the wisdom of what her son was doing, to believe that he had a purpose even if she didn't understand it. That enabled her to join him in his world for the first time. "I was giving the message that I don't need to change you. Show me who you are. I want to know. When they sense that safety, that love, and that acceptance, they have the opportunity to find their own motivation to choose whether they want to be with us or not."

Caleb chose to be with his mother. Joy says she constantly got the message from her son that he wanted to get better.

Joy was so inspired by their early success with the program that she wanted to give Caleb more. By then the mother of two younger girls, both neurotypical, she only had time to spend about ten hours a week in the room with Caleb, even though she was homeschooling him. But she wanted more.

She went to her church with a plea for help. Five people agreed to let her train them in the Son-Rise approach and to spend time in the room with Caleb. Others agreed to watch her younger children while she spent time in the room. Together they were able to give Caleb thirty-five hours of one-on-one room time a week—time that neurotypical people were spending in Caleb's world.

All this one-on-one validation of Caleb's experiences allowed him to feel safe coming further and further out of his shell. He started to show his winning personality. "He's the type of kid that people look at because anything excites him," Joy says. "He gets excited about the smallest things. People are drawn to that, intoxicated by that. I wish I would get that excited about life."

About six months later, Joy introduced academics to the room, teaching Caleb what his peers were learning in first and second grade at school.

"I'm not ready for school," Caleb told her when this began. He said, "In 2010 I will be ready for school and then my autism will be gone." He was still so far behind that she didn't believe him.

But Joy was learning as much in that room as Caleb was.

"Choosing to accept him where he's at, I learned really how to love," she says. "I don't want to sound like parents who don't do this, don't love their children, because I hadn't done it till he was eight and I thought I loved him. [But] this gave me an opportunity to say: *It's not Caleb having autism that's causing my frustration, my level of stress. It's how I'm choosing to look at it, to perceive it—that's what's affecting my stress level and my emotional state.*"

As Caleb's comfort level increased, he was able to handle two adults in the room with him at once, both tuning in to him, and then three people at a time. Then Joy started bringing in kids his own age to spend time with Caleb in the room. By the summer of 2010, eighteen months after her first Son-Rise training, Caleb could handle three children in the room with him at once, and Joy realized he had been right—he would be ready for third grade in the fall, just one school year behind.

Deeply religious, Joy thanks God for guiding her to the Son-Rise Program—and helping her get a scholarship to attend the second and third training sessions. Her prayers have been answered, she says. "A year and eight months is a small price to get what we're getting today. It's not even a price to pay, really, because I've learned so much. Now, rather than Caleb having been a challenge, a burden, 'why us?'—I'm so glad it was us."

In the next chapter I will walk you through the story of another family that got extraordinary results from the many different ways they tried to help their son.

KEEP IN MIND

- Addressing behavior problems through behavioral therapies is necessary and important but usually not sufficient to thoroughly overcome autism symptoms.
- Body problems can be hidden causes of behavior problems.
- Brain problems can be hidden causes of behavior problems.
- Sensory problems can be hidden causes of behavior problems.
- As Dr. Edward C. Carr said, "Fix contexts, not behaviors."

But also remember

- There is no single thing that can fix autism.
- Medical treatments are not a substitute for behavioral approaches.
- Combining medical and behavioral therapies can often be more effective than either alone.
- No single behavioral approach is best for everyone at all times.
- You can unconditionally love your child no matter how their therapies are going.

CHAPTER 8

- - - - - - - - - - - - - - - -

From Autistic to Extraordinary

At age seventeen, Daniel Berg asked his parents whether he had once been autistic. They had been leading him to that question in preparation for a conversation with me for this book, but it was the first time he'd asked it directly. Yes, they told him, you used to be on the spectrum, but not anymore.

Today, as Daniel prepares to graduate from high school, the person he was in elementary school seems almost unrecognizable.

"I guess I was just a very strange kid," he told me. "I just remember the world being very confusing and I had a hard time interacting with people. . . . It was like I was a different person back then."

Daniel was born five weeks premature and he was a "skinny, scrawny little kid who screamed a lot," his mother, Melody Park, says. He had no obvious food allergies, but "whenever he got near food smells, he would vomit." So his diet through age ten consisted of the only things that didn't make him barf: milk, cheese, pasta, bread, ice cream, and other desserts. His only vegetables were french fries; his only fruit, apple juice.

Through the first few grades of elementary school, Daniel was extremely sensitive to loud sounds and went through a series of repetitive behaviors. He picked his nose, flapped his hands, and sucked on his shirt. He threw tantrums regularly and couldn't "roll with the punches." If his schedule was changed unpredictably, he was a mess. He went through a series of obsessions: musical instruments—he could name about one hundred by age two—then audio speakers, airplanes, the history of flight, rockets, and finally, space.

Daniel was a first child, and because he was so obviously bright, his parents thought he was just unique. When a preschool teacher told them he belonged in the special education class next door, they switched preschools.

But eventually it became obvious that their son's unusual behavior was a problem. He had no friends. He couldn't play even simple sports. He didn't seem to understand that his classmates were sick of listening to him talk about his latest obsession. Daniel was also struggling academically. He wasn't reading by the end of first grade. And he couldn't draw a straight line on a piece of paper, because he couldn't feel the pressure of the pen on the paper.

That's when Daniel's parents began, in his words, "carting him off to a variety of therapists."

Daniel's Journey

In this chapter I'm going to give you an in-depth look at Daniel's path from klutzy, odd, tantrum-prone preschooler to poised, creative, successful high school graduate. I think it's instructive to explore what his parents did to help him and what Daniel did to help himself. His story may not be directly relevant to your own. Your child may be on a different point on the spectrum. You will almost definitely have to try different strategies than his family did. (As the saying goes: If you know one child with autism, you know one child with autism.)

But Daniel's story also illustrates some of the underlying principles I've been outlining in this book that can help everyone with autism and their families:

- meet your child where he is and truly appreciate that place;
- don't underestimate your child's innate ability to improve once blockages are out of the way;
- pay attention to both body and mind;
- nurture her creativity;

- remain open to transformation;
- and finally, your unconditional love really does make a big difference.

A lot of what Daniel's parents did was to minimize his stress—both physical and emotional. They taught him to understand himself and his body. They taught him how to negotiate the neurotypical world, making it less scary and overwhelming. They taught him to appreciate himself and his gifts. All these things helped reduce Daniel's stress, helping his whole web, including his brain and body, allowing him to function to his extraordinary potential.

Most of Daniel's treatments were largely paid for by insurance, though of course there were copays, summer programs, and, for a few years, the cost of private school to provide a more sheltered environment for him. Since he turned twelve, their only expenses have been those typical for middle-class families: after-school sports, summer classes, music lessons.

"I think [Daniel] doesn't have a lot of memory of all the difficulties and how much of a struggle it was," Melody says. "I don't think he was that aware of how on the spectrum he was, and that's fine."

In the last few chapters I gave you a framework for constructively handling your child's existing limitations and challenges. I asked you to appreciate that your child is, as Daniel was before age ten, in many ways fragile and vulnerable, close to falling apart, easily overwhelmed. In this chapter I'd like to use his example to help you develop a vision for reducing that vulnerability—not just working around it. With this vision you will be energized to find ways to clear the path so the journey can be stronger, more direct, more sure, and more spontaneous. My goal is not to help you get your child off the autistic spectrum to become "normal." It's to help them become extraordinary, to become all they can be.

Anger Management

One of the first major problems that came up with Daniel was his tremendous meltdowns. Melody says she was completely perplexed by them until she read a book called *The Explosive Child,* by Ross Greene, which helped her come up with some strategies. She began keeping a log of Daniel's meltdowns—what time of day they happened, what events or activities preceded the meltdown, how long it had been since he'd eaten . . . Within a week or two she noticed a pattern she hadn't seen before: The tantrums always happened when it had been a while since his last meal, and when she needed him to be flexible.

"When he got hungry, he had no control over his emotions," she says. The weird thing was, he wasn't asking for food, and didn't seem to even notice that he was hungry. Melody started bringing a snack when she picked him up from school, and that seemed to help. She also discovered that when she was pressed for time and expected him to respond to her need to rush or run an errand, he couldn't. "I realized I had to go at his pace," she says.

Then, just as she thought she was getting a handle on Daniel's tantrums, he went nuclear at a sporting goods store. His grandfather had taken him to buy a sleeping bag for an overnight trip that they were both eagerly anticipating. But the store was out of blue sleeping bags and Daniel erupted when his grandfather suggested a green one instead.

It was only later, in analyzing the meltdown, that Melody realized her mistakes. Daniel was probably hungry. And he didn't seem to realize that sleeping bags came in different colors—to him, a "sleeping bag" was what they had looked up on the Internet. And that one was blue, not green. Once Melody recognized that Daniel didn't understand that the blue and green ones were the same thing, she began priming him for shopping trips. "They may not have exactly the one you want," she'd tell him. "If you don't like the ones they have, you can say 'no thank you,' and we'll keep looking."

By the time he was in first grade, his tantrums were pretty much over.

Repetitive Behaviors

The next thing to go were his tics. Because Daniel was so smart, Melody was pretty much able to talk him out of his repetitive behaviors. As soon as he would start a new one—like sucking on his shirt collar—Melody would gently remind him about the time he sucked so long and so hard that he got a neck ache. She reminded him a lot—a whole lot. After about a week of constant reminders, he stopped. This also worked with the hand flapping, which was causing early signs of carpal tunnel syndrome in his wrists. When he started obsessively sucking on his fingers, she talked about how the habit would make him sick. Finally, around age six, Daniel seemed to outgrow his need for these repetitive behaviors. Melody thinks it was the consistency of her reminders, and the fact that she jumped on new tics quickly, before they could become solid habits, that made the difference for Daniel.

Learning Issues

By the end of first grade, Daniel could talk a blue streak and had an almost adult vocabulary. But he was at the bottom of his class in reading. His teacher recommended a summer program called Reading Revolution, a multisensory course that teaches reading by grounding it in bodily experience through card games, jumping, playing ball, and other movement-based activities. He had a tutor twice a week, and by the time school started again, Daniel was reading at a sixth-grade level.

I've already mentioned the importance of whole-body involvement in learning, so it makes sense that movement helped Daniel learn. His parents were impressed by this power of movement to address Daniel's problems both intellectually and physically and it became a central theme for many of the approaches they took.

The neuropsych testing they did on Daniel that summer at the school's request (for $4,500, with only $500 reimbursed by insurance) gave Daniel's parents a clearer sense of his strengths and weaknesses, and they started addressing them one by one.

The test showed a very big split between his verbal and performance IQ. He was particularly weak at demonstrating his knowledge.

Daniel also had visual-spatial problems. He couldn't copy things down from the blackboard, which often meant he'd miss out on homework assignments written on the board. Once they figured out the problem, his teachers made accommodations for him. They allowed Daniel to get up and walk around or step outside when he needed to take a break, they made it easier for him to read his homework sheets, by putting fewer problems on a page, and they let him type his homework instead of writing it by hand.

The testing also turned up a major deficit in his ability to tap out a rhythm. He scored in the 5th percentile in one rhythm test—as low as someone with borderline brain damage.

Depression

When Daniel was about eight, Melody became concerned about his state of mind. He had started to feel bad about himself because he couldn't play sports like the other kids, and was struggling in school. He described himself as a "tree with all the higher branches but none of the lower branches" as compared to the other kids who were the other way around—they could do lots of basic things he couldn't, while he could do some advanced things that were beyond them.

He would say things like "Oh, just throw me in the street and have a car run over me," Melody said. He had fantasies of hurting himself. Once, just to see what it felt like, he cut himself. His parents quickly found him a therapist.

He saw her for more than a year, and Daniel's father, Eli, says she was very good and helpful. "She was very sensitive to his talents," Eli says, "and very respectful of his mind."

Physical Activities

Like many parents of autistic kids, Eli and Melody signed Daniel up for occupational therapy to help with his clumsiness. Daniel says he doesn't remember any specific gains from his therapy, but he loved the big Lycra swings he used to spin in, and the zip line that landed in a giant foam pit. "I had the time of my life."

Melody also made a point of trying to find a sport Daniel enjoyed. She wanted to get him the physical experiences that most kids get on their own, but that Daniel had missed. "He was very physically awkward and he felt really bad about that," Melody said. Eli is not a play-catch-in-the-yard kind of dad, so Melody hired a sports coach who met Daniel in the park every Sunday morning for a year or two and helped him at catching and throwing. Daniel never got good at it, but he did get more comfortable handling a ball. She also arranged for him to play tennis, swim—which he did well—and ski. She experimented with a few martial arts classes and finally found Bushido, which was helpful for Daniel because it focused on centering, and the teacher was very gentle. He later moved on to another form that helped with strengthening.

Outdoor activities also became important for Daniel as he neared adolescence. He loved hiking, rock climbing, biking, and kayaking, and his parents provided him with as many different opportunities to do these as they could.

Senses in Translation

Just as Brenda Smith Myles advised parents to "live out loud," Eli says one of his biggest roles in Daniel's life was to serve as translator between Daniel's sensory world and other people's. One key example involved a slingshot. In sixth grade, Daniel decided he wanted to build a giant slingshot like one he'd seen on a TV show. Eli loaded up their station wagon with two-by-sixes and quarter-inch tubing and piled them into the backyard. But when they set to work, Daniel kept breaking the heads off the screws needed to link the boards.

Anyone who has ever worked a screwdriver knows intuitively that as you turn the screw, it gets harder and harder to turn, until finally it's impossible to move, and the job is done. When the heads kept popping off, Eli realized that his son did not understand this. He couldn't feel that increasing tension and resistance—he just kept torquing the screw hard without easing up, as if it could still turn easily.

Eli noticed the sensory perception problem and explained to Daniel how screws work—not just in the abstract, but in real time, while Daniel was trying to work. Eli carefully talked Daniel through the experience of feeling the increasing tension, giving Daniel words so that he could start to differentiate out those sensations and actually pay attention to that feeling. Eli did this a number of times, patiently repeating the translation of sensations Daniel couldn't feel into words he could hear. Finally, after a few false starts, Daniel learned how to sense the growing stiffness and was able to tighten the screw without breaking it.

Eli responded to Daniel as both a father and a scientist. He was intrigued by Daniel's sensory experiences and how the boy had problems integrating information that came from different senses. Daniel could see, hear, and feel but he could not coordinate the different information his five senses were giving him about the world.

Most neurotypical people coordinate across different senses without even thinking about it. In a noisy room most of us will have an easier time hearing someone else if we can also see that person's lips—the visual information will integrate with and support what we hear. That's not the case in some kids with autism, who tend to pay extra attention to one sense at the expense of another. Either they don't get the added benefit of seeing the lips move while hearing the person talk, for instance, or they pay so much attention to reading the lips that they can't track or even hear the words.

Eli had Daniel's sensory integration ability tested at age eleven and found that the boy had a harder time when his sense of touch and hearing were stimulated simultaneously. When Daniel could hear something and feel something at the same time, neither sense worked as well. In a noisy room Daniel had trouble seeing.

He was tested again at age fourteen, after many of his autistic behaviors had faded, and this sensory gap had disappeared. His brain could fluidly interpret information from both his ears and his fingers simultaneously. It had somehow reorganized and changed itself to gain the bandwidth needed to coordinate Daniel's senses.

RESEARCH SPOTLIGHT: OUT OF SYNCH

Some autistic adults have reported that they don't look someone in the eye because they can't hear the person and look in their eyes at the same time. If you've read Portia Iversen's book *Strange Son,* you've read about experiments with her son and with another autistic then-teenager, the author Tito Rajarshi Mukhopadhyay. Neuroscientist Michael Merzenich at UC San Francisco studied Tito's reactions and discovered that he couldn't hear and see simultaneously. When Merzenich showed Tito shapes on a computer screen, Tito could identify them accurately. When Merzenich played a tone in Tito's ear, he could hear that easily. But when Merzenich played the note and showed the shape at the same time, Tito couldn't identify both unless the tone and the shape were played at least a second and a half apart—that is, his visual and auditory information were out of synch.

Theory of Perception

For many years scientists have described people with autism as lacking a "theory of mind"—they don't understand that other people's minds are different than their own. Eli thinks neurotypicals lack a "theory of perception"—we believe that because we perceive the world in a certain way, everyone else must see it the way we do, because to us "that's the way it is."

Eli learned this lesson when Daniel was seven and almost got conked on the head by a ski lift bar. Father and son were getting settled into the chairlift when Eli saw the oncoming bar and had to shove Daniel out of the way. "I said in parental fear and anger: 'Why didn't you see that?!'" Daniel was articulate enough to answer, "If I knew why I didn't see it, I would have known to see it." Eli says that was the last time he ever got angry with his son. Daniel wasn't trying to be difficult, Eli realized, it was just that he was living in a different perceptual world. Daniel wasn't "wrong" not to see something that didn't exist in his perceptual world. He simply couldn't see it.

So Eli realized he had to stop taking his own perceptual world for granted and start translating it to Daniel so the boy could perceive that world himself. Eli started narrating the neurotypical world to Daniel, to teach him the rules he couldn't intuit by himself. One time, for example, Daniel was trying to learn to write *G*'s his teacher could understand, but each one he wrote looked different. By this point Eli knew that this was not an issue of Daniel being sloppy or careless but probably because Daniel had a different goal in mind than making identical *G*'s. Eli asked if Daniel knew that he was supposed to write each letter as if it could be placed exactly on top of the sample letter. "No," Daniel answered, "I was just making *G*'s." So Eli explained that the exercise was to copy the exact shape of the letter, not just to show the meaning of the letter. Once Daniel was told the assumptions that most other kids had understood intuitively, he was able to follow the rules and write a recognizable *G*.

Eli says his passion for meditation also helped him become the "Daniel whisperer," as he puts it. The meditative habit of watching how your mind constructs your world rather than taking it for granted turned out to be great training for understanding Daniel's different view of reality. It allowed Eli to have some awareness and control of where his own focus was. He could shift his own mind from the things he thought were important to the things that were in the background to him—the sound of one's own breath, the dust bunnies in the corner, the color of light on the floor—but in the foreground to Daniel. It allowed him to see Daniel as not "bad" or "uncooperative" but as perceiving things differently.

The best thing parents can do for their autistic kids, Eli says, is learn how to see their perceptually different world and then help them identify the differences between that world and our own. "If you can't include their reality in your own, then you've got a problem, too," Eli says. It's a great gift to them to validate their world, to show them you see it, and then to use that knowledge to help them see yours.

Understanding these perceptual differences can also give you more patience with your child. Daniel's repetitive behaviors, for instance, were not done to annoy his parents. They were about gaining some control over a world that was incredibly confusing and overwhelming. Daniel wouldn't know when he had to go to the bathroom or was hungry—his body would be sending him messages, but he didn't understand what they were saying. Daniel turned to his obsessions to block out the noise of these confusing signals. He tried to regulate his body's needs by taking audio speakers apart, not understanding that he wasn't addressing the real problem.

Eli says he used to walk down the street with Daniel and realize that Daniel had lost the mental picture of his father—as babies "lose" an object once it is taken out of their sight. Once Eli figured that out, it made sense that Daniel would often become gripped by fear walking down the street.

Of course, playing this kind of role for your child involves more than just incredible patience and commitment. It also requires boundless love for this small person in front of you, and endless fascination with every nuance, every detail—*but without judgment.*

Do your best to be totally in the moment with your child, creating a place of trust and safety, so they can transcend their own anxiety and experience the splendor of the world as they perceive it. Then they too can become fascinated and see, as William Blake put it, "a world in a grain of sand." You might find, too, that your child's world is fascinating. *Anxiety often comes from a disconnect between what your child can do and what others expect of them, and it is an obstacle to learning.* This is true for everyone, of course, but an autistic child has a lower threshold than most. The more you fall in love with your child's fascinating world, the more comfortable you get in his room, the more comfortable he can get in yours.

Eli was incredibly good at living in Daniel's world, at validating that world and at translating for Daniel the differences between his world and the one most of us perceive.

Eli was also good at hiring people, like the therapist, who could do the same. I think the tone that Eli and Melody set in Daniel's childhood

HOW TO FIND A GOOD SPECIALIST

In every specialty, there's a huge range of quality from the true master to the hack practitioner. It's tough to tell them apart based on a website or a diploma on the wall, but the difference could be life-altering for your child.

You can start checking out a potential therapist or doctor by searching their name on the Web. Check your state's licensing boards to make sure the person has not been sanctioned, as well as for reviews of their competency and quality.

Think about the process like a blind date: You need to like the other person, and they need to respect what you have to say. A doctor who tells you she knows everything and you should just do what she says is probably not the most open-minded.

How well do they listen to you? A doctor who interrupts constantly and doesn't seem to hear what you're saying is probably not a good one, regardless of her fancy résumé. For the most part you're on your own here. Friends' recommendations can help, but really, it's about trust. Do you trust the person on the other side of the exam table or desk to partner with you to help your child? Will the person believe what they see rather than hearing what they believe?

Another test is whether the person can speak articulately and with clarity about his or her work. Not everyone has the gift of language, but if a therapist can explain what he was thinking when he did something, or why this activity fits her underlying philosophy, they're likely to be better than average.

I am biased toward specialists who listen, think clearly, and are committed to helping out.

helped their son negotiate adolescence, getting better through this sometimes rocky period, rather than worse.

Eli was clear that his goal was not to make his son neurotypical, but to open up channels of communication and then allow Daniel's development to find its own creative path.

Building Integration

Eli also got Daniel working with a Feldenkrais practitioner. The Feldenkrais Method is a mind-body technique developed in the twentieth century by a Russian-born Israeli scientist and martial artist named Moshé Feldenkrais. Practitioners use gentle, but directed, touch and small movements to help clients become more aware of their bodies and to use them more efficiently. It's a way of using the body to train the brain.

Feldenkrais believed that movement is the foundation of learning. Neuroscientist Michael Merzenich told me he thinks these ideas make sense, because "the brain is thinking and feeling while it's moving. Nowhere in the brain are these things separated or occurring independently." Feldenkrais used small movements because it's easier to notice things more exquisitely when you're moving slowly, and you give your nervous system new and delicate ways of experiencing the world.

A baby who has difficulty coordinating movement won't be able to fully explore her world. A neurological problem may cause the movement problem, or vice versa, but both lead to more neurological problems and more movement problems. Because Daniel was awkward physically, he shied away from the playground games and sports that taught his friends how to gain more control over their bodies. This left him even further behind. We've got another of our vicious circles here.

Engaging the body of a person with autism can help them learn. When Daniel's parents encouraged him to play catch on weekends, or swim, or do martial arts, they were encouraging him to use his body in different ways. But they weren't pressuring him. The outcome didn't matter. They didn't need him to win. They didn't care how many balls he caught or how fast he swam or whether he got a black belt. What mattered was that he was moving his body through space, feeling it in a way that did not come as naturally to him as it does to most children.

Feldenkrais work, by encouraging gentle movements, does the same thing. I have also heard of people getting fabulous results with yoga and by getting involved with pets and service animals that encourage manageable sensory experiences and exploration. The key is to get your child moving in a way that doesn't feel threatening or stressful, but safe and comfortable. Eli aimed to open channels of communication so Daniel's creative development could start to flow. Similarly, getting any body blockages out of the way and encouraging your child to explore the physical world can open up new avenues of physical (and brain) development. Try slowing down with your child so you can grow, too!

Daniel says now, "I can't pinpoint the time when I stopped having to think about how to move my body and it became intuitive." But once it did become fluid, Daniel was able to open himself up to even more learning.

DIFFERENTIATING: MAKING DISTINCTIONS

In preparing to write this book, I had several long conversations with an impressive woman named Anat Baniel. Anat learned the Feldenkrais Method from Moshe Feldenkrais himself but has moved it along so far that she now considers her work her own. The Anat Baniel Method uses sensory and motor experience to refine and deepen experience. Anat, who specializes in treating children with special needs, feels that many people (not just those with autism) experience their bodies and sensations in large chunks and don't have much awareness of more subtle sensations or movements.

She described for me a recent lesson with a three-year-old boy who wasn't toilet trained and didn't seem to notice when his diaper was soiled. Anat took two washcloths, wetting one with warm tap water and gently rubbing it against his face.

"That's a wet towel," she told him. Then she rubbed his face with the dry one and explained the difference. She had him close his eyes and she rubbed first one, then the other, and he guessed correctly which was which. Then, with his and his mother's permission, she did the same thing with the washcloths on his bottom. He "got" that there was a difference that he had never noticed before. That was the last time he wet his pants.

Her goal, she said, was not to get him potty trained, but to *feel the difference* between wet and dry. Once the child could differentiate the two sensations, he could train himself. If he couldn't feel the difference, no amount of "training" would really work.

Anat's theory is that children with autism don't perceive distinctions, say, between themselves and the rest of the world, which is why they have trouble identifying what hurts or when they have to go to the bathroom. They are also clumsy because they can't "differentiate" the sensations in their bodies, so their senses aren't helping enough to guide their motor activity or build a foundation for their learning.

The therapist in chapter 6 was intuitively helping to differentiate when she put the tongue depressor into a child's mouth to help him feel how his moving tongue changed his sounds. Perhaps Stuart would have noticed his appendicitis and Judy would have noticed her pneumonia earlier if they had had this sensory and motor training.

The first things we learn in life are through our sensory and motor systems. Anat sees physical sensation and movement as the foundation for training the brain to make distinctions at any point in life.

By tuning people with autism in to their own nervous systems, Anat has opened the way for many to learn to speak coherently, to write and read effectively, to move gracefully, and to relate spontaneously—through her work on apparently unrelated areas of movement and action. Once the brain can differentiate among these movements and actions, it learns how to differentiate in other areas, too.

Food Issues

Melody and Eli never addressed Daniel's self-restricted "beige" diet directly. They were relieved that he would eat anything at all and they never considered trying an elimination diet.

But food and smells were a huge problem for Daniel. He got a reputation at school for barfing, and the teachers used to give him a seat near the door to help dissipate any smells that might set him off. The throwing up diminished by fourth or fifth grade, but his diet still consisted mostly of bread and cheese.

It was a five-day kayaking trip at age eleven that transformed Daniel as an eater. Melody warned him that he might not be able to eat his normal diet on the trip, and he said he wanted to go anyway. When he came back he was eating more foods. Perhaps all the physical activity made him aware of his hunger for the first time, or his sensory work was toning down his reactions, or he'd outgrown his smell sensitivities, or he was having too much fun to think about it and there was nothing else to eat anyway. Whatever got him over the hump, the trip was the beginning of Daniel's willingness to try a wide range of foods. Today, he says, his friends consider him a human garbage can because of his appetite and ability to eat anything. Incidentally, it was also at age eleven that Daniel lost the chubbiness of childhood and slimmed down.

Though Melody and Eli didn't think much of these dietary changes at the time, I wonder if his earlier eating pattern didn't contribute in some significant way to his problems and if his diet change wasn't a component of his transformation. Perhaps some vitamin or nutrient deficiencies were involved in his problems, and they dissipated when his diet normalized. Perhaps he had been having problems from all the gluten and casein without realizing it. Perhaps he was building on a positive cycle—instead of a vicious one. He'd already developed enough physical confidence to take the trip, and his sensory problems were already receding.

By eliminating the gluten and dairy obsession in favor of a more varied diet, Daniel opened himself not just to more diverse foods but to yet more new signals from the world. At the same time, the extra drag on his system that might have come from his prior diet could go away.

It was about this time that Daniel says he calmed down and became less fidgety. The dietary changes could easily have helped this along, but so could other things in the cycle. In the fullness of Daniel's story, all these efforts were linked together.

Social Growth

Seventh grade was a big transition time for Daniel. He met a boy who is still one of his closest friends. Suddenly the knowledge he'd gained through all his obsessions seemed cool to his peers, instead of boring. He got involved in the tech crew for school plays. All his years of being obsessed with speakers and other electronic gizmos now became socially relevant. "He found little niches where his abilities were appreciated," Melody said.

Daniel says he thinks he also decided to make friends. Before that, maybe he just wasn't interested in other people, and didn't value what they had to say. "Making a few close friends and doing [social] stuff outside of school made me more open to new experiences and doing cool things," he says. "I was developing a greater sense of myself and developing new skills."

His parents were also hammering him on manners. "I could be rude, not really anticipating how what I would say would affect others," Daniel admits. This was another area where his mother and father carefully narrated and translated between his world and the neurotypical one. His parents and therapists called attention to these behaviors and explained why other people might take offense at them. But the grown-ups didn't stop there; they also had him role-play to go through proper social behaviors. They gave him lots of concrete help in understanding and practicing new ways of relating. "I'm still trying to behave better to people," Daniel said.

Creative Juices Flow

A drum set also changed Daniel's life. When he was twelve, he went to the home of one of his father's colleagues. While the adults worked, Daniel messed around on the man's drum set. By the end of the day he was hooked.

"I found the place where the rhythm comes from inside of me," he says. "Once I locked into the beat, the pathways necessary to do that became forged in my mind."

He built himself an electronic drum set and later graduated to a "real" one. This kid who had scored nearly "brain damaged" in finger tapping as a five-year-old was becoming an accomplished drummer.

Daniel picked up guitar in late elementary school and started getting seriously into bluegrass music. In a band, he made friends. "Music has given me personal growth and helped me reconnect with my physical ability and with my soul," Daniel says.

Also while in eighth grade, he discovered drawing, and quickly developed an artistic style. Now, he says, it's evolved into a visual repertoire. Daniel's drawings are detailed and precise, with layers of muscles and tubes. His lines are long and sinuous and parallel—just the type of controlled marks he would have been unable to make six or seven years earlier, when he couldn't figure out how much pressure to apply to a pen to even draw a line at all.

The drawing has trained him and also freed him to express new things. His earlier fascination with rockets and robots now comes out in his drawings.

Now, he says, his inner rhythm shows through in many forms. "I can express [this rhythm] through art, or my mandolin or beat boxing or talking," he says. "Being connected with that has given me a thing that I can always connect to, that will be with me till the day I die. That's just what every creative person experiences in their lives. It gave me a motivation to get better."

Rhythms can help the brain better organize itself. The brain's own signaling system is based on electrical rhythms, and music and other arts can engage those rhythms. These rhythmic patterns help organize perception and experience in many domains beyond the arts themselves. Rhythms are at play when people are "in synch" with one another—rhythms of speech, of breathing, of gestures, of pace of words, of nuance, and more. They can also, as we see with Daniel, boost self-confidence and social inclusion.

People with autism can have an edge over neurotypicals in art because of their unusual view of the world. June Groden says her students make fantastic photographers because they focus on images that neurotypicals miss. Their images aren't just impressive for someone who is autistic, she says, but impressive for anyone—and that helps build self-esteem, and sales. Photography and many other artistic skills are also often manageable regardless of severe physical disabilities. Groden says one of the most talented photographers she's ever seen is deaf and has Down syndrome. Is it those "deficits" that give him a compelling and unique eye on the world? Or is it that distinctive ways of perceiving are strengths rather than deficits?

Eli says the same of Daniel's music and art and his approach to life—they're all more distinctive because of his history.

Emotions in Tune

It wasn't that Daniel lacked emotions. He could laugh or cry or get angry. But emotions weren't meaningful to him. He couldn't name them. He didn't really know what to make of the tears that might be streaming out of his eyes or the tightness in his chest. If you can barely notice that you have to pee, how are you going to notice that you are sad, happy, or angry? How do you know you need to communicate something if you don't even know you're feeling it?

For most of us, if we're watching a horror film and our heart starts to race, we have a pretty good idea why. But Daniel didn't link the physical sensations with "emotions." This disconnection from emotions probably made the world seem scarier and more confusing, Eli says.

Five days of sitting still at a meditation retreat taught Daniel, then fifteen, how to feel.

"Through meditation, I was able to consolidate my emotions into definable and understandable experiences and take a significant leap in terms of my own self-knowledge," Daniel says. He realized for the first time that each emotion had a template of physical feeling associated with it. When you are happy about something, you smile and you feel warm and bubbly. When you're sad, your face sags and you feel heavier.

It was around this time that Daniel says he "transcended" autism. "I was no longer impaired in the sense that I didn't feel so much encumbered in a social context." The eccentricities and eclectic behaviors became a sense of humor and joy for himself and others.

Lessons Learned

It's impossible to know what made the fundamental difference for Daniel, what allowed him to reduce his stress and move off the spectrum. It might have been simply the act of growing up. Autism can be described as a "developmental delay." Maybe he just developed late and caught up. Certainly it helped that Daniel was smart and curious and wanted to be a part of the world his friends inhabited. I suspect that though these things were all part of it, what let him truly "transcend autism" was the combination of most or all of the things his parents did.

Even as we celebrate his achievements, we will never know exactly what made Daniel's transformative growth possible. The only way to know what really makes a difference for kids with autism is to do a better job of studying them as they try to reconnect and feel better, and what happens along the way.

"A lot of what were huge issues now make him a very spontaneous, creative, interesting guy," Eli says. "Daniel has some elements that stick out a little, but they're not jagged anymore, they're not cutting anymore. They're making him interesting."

In the next chapter I will set forth a challenge and a request. I'm asking you to join the Autism Revolution.

KEEP IN MIND

- Profound transformation is possible.
- Narrating the neurotypical world can help people with autism better understand it. The reverse is true as well.
- Getting body problems out of the way makes it easier to be extraordinary.
- Interests that start as narrow obsessions can become rich resources for skills, creativity, and relationships.
- You can be extraordinary and autistic at the same time.
- Connecting is not just about relating to other people. It's also about connecting to inner sources of creativity.
- Everyone deserves and needs unconditional love no matter what state they're in; learning flows best when people feel safe and are seen for who they are.

But remember

- You don't have to totally get over autism or other problems to be extraordinary.
- There is no single best way of being.

CHAPTER 9

Lead the Revolution!

Looking back, Carol Connolly says it was the high-powered pediatric gastroenterologist who turned her into a revolutionary.

"Your son's autistic. Autistic kids are just this way," the doctor told her when she asked for help with Stuart's chronic diarrhea. The five-year-old just needed a little more roughage in his diet, plus some yogurt, the doctor said.

On the drive home, Carol turned on the radio and happened to hear autism advocate and mom Karyn Seroussi talking about how much the gluten-free, casein-free diet had helped her child.

Carol kept turning these two different visions of treatment around in her head—the hopelessness of the doctor's and the potential of the mother's. And the doctor's just didn't ring true. Stuart was already eating two bunches of bananas, a gallon of orange juice, and a box of Triscuits every day. How much more fiber could be stuffed into his tiny body?

"I came home and [decided] I'm going to try the exact opposite of what this guy told me to do."

Instead of adding yogurt, she cut all dairy out of her son's diet.

Stuart, who had flat-out refused to potty train, "started using the bathroom in the space of a week."

Emboldened by her success (and the horrific sounds that were still coming out of her son's bathroom), Carol decided she needed to do more. She went to her pediatrician, saying she planned to take gluten out of Stuart's diet and wanted to make sure he'd still get proper nutrition. "You're crazy," the pediatrician told her. Will it harm him? she asked. No, the pediatrician said, but getting rid of gluten will be a nightmare and a waste of time, he said. Don't bother.

She did it anyway.

And again Stuart seemed to respond well.

That was it. There was no turning back. Carol was now convinced that she knew as much about taking care of Stuart as the so-called experts did. She would listen to them in the future, but she wasn't going to let them lead the battle. She was taking control.

"As soon as you get a good result, you have to keep going," Carol says now. "Every step of the way I had incontrovertible evidence that I was doing something that was having some kind of [positive] impact on my child."

What We Need to Know and Don't

As you may have gathered by now, one of the big problems with treating autism is that we don't have enough information about what works and what doesn't, what's worth spending your time and money on and what's a waste of both. Making it even harder is that people with autism can be so different from each other. This is a *spectrum of spectrums.* Every level, every part of the web I've told you about has a variety of ways of presenting itself. There are a number of ways of having a disturbed immune or digestive system; dozens of paths to mitochondrial problems, sensory troubles, and injuries; hundreds of possible genetic mutations; all manner of behaviors; and many thousands of potentially dangerous environmental exposures.

Even more, each person might have different symptoms and needs at different times in their life. A treatment that fails someone at one point may work for the same person at a later one. Perhaps there was a metaphorical big rock in the way on the first try, but if other treatments remove the rock, a second or third try may work amazingly well.

You can see from this why it would be virtually impossible to solve all your child's problems once and for all. Even if you achieve great success, you will still need to be on the lookout for dangers that might erode your child's health. You and your child will have to remain vigilant to protect against toxins, maintain a superhealthy diet, avoid bugs, and keep stress as low as possible. The hills under the lake may still be there, even if you've gotten the water level to rise.

You didn't deserve autism, and I'm sure there are times you wish it weren't part of your life, but it is an ongoing commitment for you and your whole family. My saying this isn't meant to discourage you—quite the opposite. By acknowledging that beating back autism is a long-term commitment, I hope to save you from getting discouraged by the inevitable setbacks.

Many people will get involved in helping your child. That's a gift for them as well as for you. The people who volunteered to help Caleb had experiences that transformed their career paths and changed their lives, Joy says.

I think that as a society and a species, we're facing a new situation with autism (and other chronic conditions, too). We have never had to deal with so many young people whose potential is limited by autism and other learning and behavioral disabilities (1 out of 6 children total!), so many childhood allergies, so many older adults hobbled by Parkinson's and Alzheimer's, so much cancer, and so many people in middle age coping with autoimmune problems. It's all the more concerning if my strong suspicion proves correct—that these are largely acquired conditions, not inevitable ones.

Lots to Love

Autism can bring with it a lot of physical pain and suffering. Between the diarrhea, seizures, sleep disorders, social anxieties, sensory issues, language problems, clumsiness, repetitive behaviors, and general sense of feeling "different," there are a lot of undesirable aspects to autism. The low adult employment is also a huge problem, and makes full independence a long shot.

But of course there are lots of things to treasure about the autistic mind, too.

There are the incredible insights and creativity that come from a different perspective on the world, and the distinct way their senses allow them to perceive it. The artistic talents of people with autism run the gamut from photography to music composition, set design to glass blowing.

There's the intellect and attention to detail. A lot of our universities, corner offices, and top government posts are filled with people on the high-functioning end of the spectrum. Though their social skills may be below average, their brainpower more than compensates. Many of our greatest innovations wouldn't have happened without people with autism.

For Carol Connolly, what's most endearing about Stuart is his warm personality. "He's a really sweet kid," she said, especially when he's not in pain. "We're very lucky in that we have a child who is so emotionally engaged and rewarding. He gives us so much back."

Daniel is obviously going to contribute a tremendous amount to the world through his intellect and his musical and creative abilities.

Jimmy and Caleb are headed for full lives, unlimited by autism's problems.

The future is still uncertain for little Crystal, but at least she's feeling better and is getting easier to parent.

Ana Todd is planning a career change. She wants to put to work everything she's learned from having autism and chronic fatigue. She's now studying for medical school entrance exams and working on building her health enough to get pregnant.

And Judy Endow, who still has autism, is making a big difference in the lives of people with autism through her consulting, writing, and speaking—as well as helping neurotypicals "get" what autism is about.

Pain and Resilience

An autism diagnosis has a huge emotional impact for almost everyone. It is not something you can prepare for. You may have hopes and dreams that feel shattered. Our healthcare and school systems are also unprepared for the current flood of complicated, high-need, and hard-to-handle people. The general public only sees the surface behaviors, doesn't understand what's really going on, and is quick to make uninformed judgments.

For Carol Connolly, one of the hardest things to accept is how similar Stuart is to so many other family members, and yet "this kid got it one hundred times worse." Where Carol's siblings can use their Asperger's-like qualities to succeed in careers like engineering and chemistry, her son struggles with basic self-control.

Many people are upset by the possiblility that environmental factors may have contributed to their child's autism. In the United States, we were all raised to think that our government protects us from dangerous products. It may come as a shock to realize that many everyday chemicals are not well tested, and that the government doesn't always work in our best interest. Taking in this information is a big adjustment, and anger is a natural reaction.

Please understand that you can be a total bulldog about getting what your child truly needs but still act with compassion toward the many players in the healthcare and school systems. Just as you look for teaching moments with your child, you can look for teaching moments with these professionals, helping them understand your child and how they can help.

Watch out for anger or other pain that distracts you from being fully present and loving with your child. Your child needs your full presence and love to keep anxiety down and health-promoting processes moving along well.

The diagnosis is what it is. You have the power to transform its meaning as well as its outcome. Even with all the pain, huge numbers of parents find new camaraderie and purpose in learning innovative ways to love and make a difference in the world.

You Need to Be in Charge; but You Need Help, Too

The fact is that *you* need to be in charge of your child's treatment. As much as you want a doctor, therapist, alternative medicine practitioner, or teacher to tell you how to "fix" your child, that's not likely to happen.

Covering all the territory in this book has reminded me how hard it is to know enough to make a difference in autism. Some of what makes it difficult is training—it's tough to find people who have a comprehensive understanding of autism along with a detailed knowledge of everything from allergies to gut bugs, neurons to tantrums. Some of it is philosophy: People often believe that their part of the proverbial elephant is the whole elephant. Each doctor and caregiver can help in the areas they know best, in the limited time that insurance constraints allow. There are too few specialists who know how to guide you and your child through a long and complex journey to untangle their troubled web.

You—as well as your spouse, if you are lucky—will usually be the only one capable of seeing your whole child. You must be your child's facilitator, translator, medic, nutritionist, scientist, and mom or dad all wrapped into one. Carol Connolly and her husband continue to play these roles for Stuart. As do Eli Berg and Melody Park for Daniel, Cindy Franklin for Jimmy, Nell and Eric Kubik for Crystal, and Joy and Christian Petersen for Caleb. As adults, Ana Todd and Judy Endow must be their own advocates.

All of these people I've introduced to you also have another thing in common: They've found ways to collaborate with at least some of the doctors and therapists they've met, even ones who don't "get" the whole picture. Carol Connolly had to go outside mainstream medicine to find some of the information that has made the biggest difference for Stuart. Even so, she long ago decided to educate her mainstream doctors, so they would be more open-minded the next time a patient with autism came along. "I had this idea that if what we were doing [with Stuart] was the right thing, then we needed to bring the medical establishment with us," Carol says. "If this is working, science is going to catch up with me, and I want to be there when they figure it out."

That's why she still goes to the same pediatrician who told her she was crazy for cutting gluten out of Stuart's diet. He apologized when he saw how much Stuart improved, and now invites her in every year to explain to him what she's learned. "I felt like I owed it to the other parents in the practice to have him follow Stuart," Carol says, "in the hopes that the next family wasn't going to hit the [same] wall."

Carol says she now calls her son's longtime doctors by their first names—and considers them members of Stuart's team. She has her expertise and they have theirs. "I want to make sure there's a partnership and a dialogue there where my concerns are being heard, and they're giving me the science back in a way that I can use it.

"I want the benefit of their training, but they need the benefit of my experience."

Why Medicine Needs the Autism Revolution

Autism presents many challenges to medical practice. Because it's a "spectrum of spectrums"—with many parts of the web, and differences between people with autism at every one of those parts—it is hard to study. It's also hard to treat. These days specialists usually deal with only one thing, and general practitioners have very little time to give each patient. So how do you deal with a whole web of interlocking issues?

In "evidence-based medicine" research you collect a group of people who are as similar as possible, and then test them on a single treatment, while keeping everything else the same. But how can you collect a group of people with autism who are truly similar? Even if everyone has autism behaviors, they probably are different from one another in their genes, cells, guts, immune systems, and brains. They probably eat differently and have different stressors. And how can you keep everything else the same? Parents are often unwilling to maintain the status quo, because the current state of affairs is so challenging, and because they feel they don't have any time to waste. And each person may be delicately enough balanced that they themselves may be different from one day to the next.

What does this mean? First, saying that a treatment works or doesn't work for autism often overlooks that it may truly work for 20 percent even though it doesn't work for the other 80 percent—because the success gets washed out in the averaging. Second, studying treatments one at a time doesn't help you or your doctors determine which particular complex set of treatments is optimal for your particular child, or how to make the frequent adjustments that may be needed.

As new genetic and systems biology discoveries pile up, scientists, doctors, and all of us are humbled by how complex most medical disorders are. Even PKU, the enzyme dysfunction we discussed in chapter 2, which was once thought to be a single gene condition, is now seen as much more complicated. Not only are there well over five hundred different kinds of PKU mutations, but the PKU gene works in connection with each person's own unique genome. Charles Scriver, a world-renowned pediatrician and geneticist, says that every patient has her own complex way of having PKU, and should be treated accordingly.

The Autism Revolution is about the same sort of paradigm shift.

Treatment Successes Are an Untapped Scientific Gold Mine

If we had no idea that anyone with autism could get better, maybe it would make sense to work "bottom up," one treatment at a time, to find things that make it budge even a little. It would be worth the wait.

But people with autism *are* getting better, right now, with resources and knowledge we already have, often by working on many different parts of the web at one time. *Under duress, you and parents like you are performing remarkable natural experiments in pulling your children back from the brink.*

Not every person with autism who goes down this road makes it all the way. Some achieve modest success and others achieve little or none. But the mere existence of progress is big news. I believe that the efforts families are making to get their kids better, and especially the very successful efforts, are a remarkable untapped gold mine of valuable data.

In this book I've had to piece together information from each different part of the web. A true systems biology approach would look at all these levels at the same time to see how they really interact. Right now we have lots of dots. We don't have much research to draw lines to connect even two of those dots. Going forward, we need to map the real web using the most sophisticated measurement technologies we have.

Let's take food. Most studies of diet and autism try to see whether diet changes autistic behaviors. And many researchers who conduct this research believe the answer will be no. But we've seen that the answer is often yes. And in children where the diet has helped, many families report a large number of changes, well beyond behavior. Changing a child's diet may . . .

- Change cells by:
  - Changing nutrients involved in molecular and metabolic processes
  - Changing the lipid profile, which changes cell membranes and molecular signals
- Change the digestive system by:
  - Starving out some kinds of gut bugs and giving others food they like better
  - Changing by-products from bugs and the immune system that may impact the brain

- Achieving toilet training
- Getting rid of bad breath
- Change stimuli to the immune system, which may help by:
  - Getting rid of rashes
  - Reducing or eliminating allergic reactions
  - Improving sleep
  - Reducing inflammation, which can reduce irritation of brain sensory processing systems
- Change the child's brain by:
  - Improving brain cell health
  - Improving brain blood flow
  - Sometimes reducing seizure severity or frequency
  - Increasing signal and reducing noise in sensory processing
  - Strengthening brain network coordination
  - Expanding the child's sensory experience
- Change behavior by:
  - Reducing irritability and jumpy behavior
  - Reducing aggression
  - Expanding the child's sensory universe by engaging the child in food
  - Increasing alertness
  - Prolonging attention span
  - Reducing impulsiveness
  - Improving language frequency and complexity
  - Improving eye contact
  - Improving relatedness and communication
- Change gene expression by:
  - Increasing nutrients that support DNA repair mechanisms
  - Decreasing substances that could lead to DNA-damaging processes like oxidative stress
  - Promoting healthier gene expression
- Make more room for the extraordinary by:
  - Removing distraction and drag on the brain
  - Letting all the systems that support the brain do a much better job

And probably lots more.

At present there is no autism diet study that looks at virtually any of this except for a few behavioral items. And if you don't study it, how do you map it all together as a systems biology web? Yet all of this is going on all at once in a small child who starts on a new diet. If our children's bodies can handle this, our science should be able to handle it, too.

Whole-Body Autism Science: Studying Complex Treatments over Time

We know that few if any people with autism are likely to experience major transformation from any one treatment. It usually takes a combination of many things over time. And we know that different things work for different people. So, how can we study this scientifically?

This needs **systems biology,** which means studying things as they interact, rather than looking at them separately.

The explosion of computer speed, data analysis techniques, portable data collection devices (like your cellphone), and lab equipment that

ARE REACTIONS THAT LOOK OR FEEL BAD ALWAYS DANGEROUS?

How do you tell the difference between a bad reaction and a transition your child's body needs to make? Ana Todd went through two weeks of poor coordination and greatly increased clumsiness while her brain "recalculated" as she was starting her medical treatments. Then she emerged with much more fluid and stronger movement.

Killing off infectious bugs, such as the millions of parasites Stuart's gastro-enterologist found, can lead to a temporary "die-off reaction" (sometimes called a Herxheimer reaction) when the bugs are dying but all their noxious junk hasn't yet been cleared from the body. This should usually go away in days to a week or two. But some reactions to drugs and food (and to toxins and bugs) can be dangerous, even life-threatening.

You can get an experienced clinician to help you tell the difference between a transition reaction and a bad or dangerous reaction.

can measure more things with smaller samples—all of this makes new and more flexible systems science possible. Whole-body autism needs these approaches. Here are some of them:

- *Single subject, repeated measures:* tracking each person over time, looking at their own rate of change, compared to themselves before. This avoids the problem of being confused by huge differences between individuals.
- *Intensive multivariate longitudinal design:* performing repeated measures over time at multiple levels of the web—gene expression, metabolism, lipids, immune system, gut bugs, brain blood flow, brain electricity, brain networks, behavior, learning, and relatedness. This allows us to look at each person's web, the configuration of each unique individual on the "spectrum of spectrums."
- New methods of *telehealth and electronic diaries:* allowing parents, caregivers, or people with autism to enter and upload data throughout the day. This allows us to track change right as it happens.
- *Wearable data monitors:* using easy-to-wear devices that can track things like stress levels. Examining factors that increase or reduce stress can lead to solutions.
- *"Omics"* like genomics, metabolomics, lipidomics, proteomics, gut microbiomics, and more: measuring thousands of things at one time. This allows us to look at broad changes that are occurring in many systems over time.
- *Dynamic brain measures:* looking at physiological measures likely to change with whole-body treatment, such as brain electrical signals, blood flow, metabolism, sensory processing, information processing, and connectivity networks. This helps us to see what cell, tissue, and information-processing functions in the brain may respond to treatment, and what body changes may go along with these brain changes. Some of these may soon be trackable with wearable data monitors.
- *Multileveled and nested statistical methods:* using approaches that can analyze intensive information, instead of only a few variables

and changes at a time. This may involve nesting (or grouping) children into doctor or therapist practices, or treatments into the body or brain systems they target.

- *Comparative effectiveness research:* comparing forms of clinical practice. If some clinical approaches get consistently better outcomes than others, they can be used as role models.
- *Community-based participatory research:* encouraging members of the community—this means you, parents and people with autism, clinicians, caregivers, and more—to partner with scientists to identify problems, determine the best ways to study them, and to carry out the study.

Reverse-Engineering Autism from Treatment Successes

Reverse-engineering means figuring out how something was built by looking at how it works. Many autistic children (and others) do this spontaneously—taking apart clocks, for example, and putting them back together.

Since we have people who get better, can we reverse-engineer "getting better" to figure out how autism "works"?

The National Institute of Mental Health is conducting such a study, of "remitted" autism. They are taking exhaustive histories from kids who are already free of their autism symptoms—including making sure they were really autistic in the first place—and then doing lab, genetic, and brain tests.

What if we did that in real time? Imagine if, when a newly diagnosed child walked into a clinician's office, we could get baseline measures and then track these changes as the child proceeds along her journey trying to get better. We could do this in a systems biology way, taking measures of many parts of the web and examining what changes and in what order.

I think that tracking these changes in the different parts of the web will tell us huge amounts about how autism works. Then the basic scientist hunting for molecular clues will have more to go on.

If we knew what the biology of recovery looked like in autism, we could go after it more surely—for autism and likely for a lot of other chronic diseases as well.

Grassroots Science for the Autism Revolution

One of the most frustrating things about battling autism is having to forge your own path. Families touched by autism can help their child as well as themselves *and* at the same time be part of making science more relevant by collecting and pooling their own data.

Families have been tracking treatment impacts for years on Listservs and in support groups. The more observant you are, the more opportunities you are likely to see for helping your child, the more aware you will be of what helps—and the more your experience will be able to help others.

When this revolution started, every family's breakthrough discovery had to be rediscovered in the house next door. Now there is a growing support structure. Keen observations by parents have inspired a growing number of important scientific studies.

How can you become a grassroots scientist?

1. Be systematic about what you do. Don't change too many things at once, because then you won't know what caused successes, or

problems. If possible, change one thing at a time—and then *observe carefully.*

2. Keep data. Track treatments, behavior, sleep, activities, and of course, food, toxins, bugs, and stress. You can do this in binders, on a computer, or online. At the end of this book you'll find forms to get you started, and a sample tracking form.

3. The Autism Research Institute has created a treatment checklist called the ATEC (Autism Treatment Evaluation Checklist) that you can use to record some of these observations. It now has some published scientific support. You can print it out or use it online.

4. Discuss data and how you solved problems. There are support groups, Listservs, workshops, and conferences for families like yours.

5. Participate in an online database and share your data. Joining an active database will probably make increasing sense as these resources mature.

6. Carefully investigate treatments and the science associated with them. You should know that with many studies, all you can read for free is the "abstract," a short summary. Sometimes libraries, universities, and advocacy groups can help you access the full study.

7. Lobby for treatment-relevant research.

8. Advocate for comprehensive whole-body autism training for doctors and all other caregivers and therapists. We need caregivers to understand how much transformation is possible, and how to collaborate with others working on different parts of the web. Even simply helping caregivers learn when to refer for appropriate care could make a huge difference.

9. Advocate to get specialists trained to provide complex, individualized treatments that evolve over time as the patient changes. Right now this training is not available in medical schools, residencies, or any other professional training programs. This training should be for a whole team—doctors, nurses, therapists, dietitians, physical and occupational therapists and so on, plus lay support people. There is so much to do, we need as many people as possible to pitch in.

Learn to read research critically. A study is only as good as its methods and assumptions. Researchers aren't always aware that their methods are weak. Learn how to look beneath the surface.

Some Things to Watch Out For

- Lumping people together who are different.
- Missing important parts of the picture. Is the study taking things out of context?
- Not understanding the "gray zone." Looking only for a huge effect, when a small one might be destructive or helpful, too.
- Confusing correlation with cause and effect. Scientists sometimes claim that one thing caused another, when in fact they just happened to occur at the same time.
- Making more of the results than the size and power of a study allows. Particularly in a condition as varied as autism, a study that has only a handful of subjects or even a few dozen should be viewed with caution. Any improvements could have happened by chance. Or they could have been real in a subgroup that was too small to affect the overall result. The risks or benefits your child faces may be far greater than what the study showed.
- Animal studies are terrific for showing how the body works: what individual genes do, and what happens when this part doesn't work right. They're not nearly as good at illustrating the effects or potential side effects of drugs, however, because mice are different from humans in so many ways.

Draw Strength from the Big Picture

An autism instruction manual will never be a recipe, and a treatment plan from a clinical trial will never be comprehensive or permanent. Whatever else you may do, you can draw strength from a framework by which you can judge for yourself whether something makes sense right now, and whether all your child's bases are covered. That's what I've given you in this book.

The framework I am suggesting starts with *reducing the total load of burden on your child wherever you can, and providing smart support when feasible.* The body is amazingly good at self-repair when it has the room and means to do so—so give it as much of what it needs as possible, and then watch what results.

Here I'm going to summarize the rest of the framework that I have presented throughout this book, to jog your memory and also help you see these ideas in a new way, now that you have the whole-body picture:

- Autism emerges from an interconnected web of accumulated problems.
- Autism emerges when the total load of difficulties exceeds what your child's brain and body can handle.
- Autism is not a predetermined and fixed path. It can change over a lifetime or a day, for better or for worse.
- Stress at any one point in the web can make it harder for other, often seemingly unconnected things to work well. Conversely, removing a stress may create a small change but it can sometimes create a healthy tipping point, giving your child's system the leeway to correct itself.
- Good nutrition and diet are essential for recovering and maintaining cell and whole-body health.
- Sometimes simple approaches work best. You don't always need a cannon to blow a hole through autism. Dietary changes and small, slow movements can make room for dramatic shifts over time.
- Even when you use big guns like strong medications, a foundation of healthy habits around food, toxins, bugs, and stress can help a lot.
- Genes create risk but you can reduce that risk by creating a healthy, low-toxin daily environment.
- Toxins are likely to be even more damaging to people with autism, because whatever made them autistic also likely makes them more vulnerable.

- Gut and immune health are key to overall health. Restore the digestive system and reduce inflammation by eating a healthy diet, avoiding allergens, looking for and eliminating infections, getting probiotics, sleeping well, and managing stress.
- Reduce sensory and social stress and avoid overload. Understand your child enough to know which environments will test her limits and try to avoid them and/or minimize their stress. Consider stress-reducing activities such as exercise, mindfulness, sensory integration, neuromotor training, body work, yoga, martial arts, and art, animal, or music therapy.
- Join your child where he is. Your child needs an ally to "get" why life is so hard for them, to translate things they don't understand and to create environments that will help them thrive.
- Don't worry about getting a specific result, just be present for your child and encourage the learning process. Find teachable moments in what they love. When they're fascinated with something, help them enrich it—not just do it again and again. Take advantage of the moment to commune with them and expand their world.
- Don't underestimate your child. Many, many (if not all) autistic people are capable of doing the extraordinary.
- Remember unconditional love.

I recommend that you cover as many of these bases, as many parts of the web as you can at any one time—*without* driving yourself crazy. When you try to learn what you need to know to be able to handle all these levels, you will have some compassion for your doctors, psychologists, and therapists, and for yourself. No one was trained to think about all these things at one time; no parent can manage them all perfectly day after day, year after year.

When your current strategies hit a blockage—when you feel your child is capable of doing more or getting better—then skilled sleuthing and testing may be able to identify the bump. A resourceful clinician can use judgment as well as science to identify the best combination and sequence of approaches to hurdle over it.

The good news is that this does become easier over time, once you have replaced more and more destructive vicious circles with regenerative, positive ones. If you're really lucky and hit the right strategies early on, the challenges of autism may only be a part of your life for a few years. If you have to search harder and try more approaches, your child might not ever reach society's definition of "ordinary." But your child doesn't have to use neurotypical words and social graces to achieve the extraordinary. Just ending his diarrhea, her seizures, and their tantrums will go a long way toward making all of your lives less frustrating and more fulfilling.

The truth is that you can't afford not to do this. Every bit of extra independence you gain for your child not only saves money but gives you more priceless peace of mind for the future.

As a society we can't afford not to do it, either. Costs of autism care are soaring while budgets are shriveling up. We need to get the best out of every dollar we spend on autism. If people can get a lot better, that not only is good for themselves and their families, but it also saves money for society.

Helping people with autism improve their health and well-being can teach us so much about handling profound environmentally related illnesses. This can help so many people with autism, and many millions more with other chronic illnesses. Learning from people with autism can give us new perspectives and new perceptions. In teaching us about themselves, people with autism may also teach us profoundly about addressing the current challenges of life on earth.

In the final chapter, I will offer suggestions for improving your whole family's—and your next child's—health.

KEEP IN MIND

- Science needs to take a fresh approach to autism.
- We need all hands on deck to solve this huge and complex challenge.
- Parents can help by being careful and meticulous observers.
- Parents, doctors, therapists, other caregivers, and people with autism all need to be part of the team together.

But remember

- You should not treat your child without medical help.
- Enjoy your child. They learn better when they feel safe, not stressed.
- Increasing the dose or frequency of a treatment isn't always better, and may often be harmful.
- Exhausting yourself doing many treatments isn't better than doing a few carefully chosen ones really well.

CHAPTER 10

Do It for Yourself, Your Next Baby, Your Family, and Your World

Waking up nauseous for the second morning in a row, Rose Blaire was pierced with panic. This wasn't food poisoning, she realized. It was pregnancy.

Rose and her husband, Lewis, had decided not to have any more kids. They adored their boys, Foster, then thirteen, and Nate, six, but both were on the autism spectrum and racked with health problems. The couple knew they couldn't handle a third child with those kinds of needs.

"We really wanted to have more children, but we saw what our other two were struggling with," Rose says. "We didn't want to take the chance of having another child with autism."

Rose knew the odds were high as someone who already had kids on the spectrum.

Within an hour of buying one of those drugstore pregnancy tests and confirming her suspicions, Rose turned to the Web and searched "preventing autism." She was determined to do whatever she could to give this baby a healthy start to life.

"It's not that I don't love my two oldest children—obviously, I do— but I see what they struggle with and I didn't want that to happen again," Rose says.

If Autism Develops

Where does autism come from? No one knows now, and we may never figure out what starts the cascade or pushes it over the tipping point. In some cases, the risk for autism may be so strong that it is like an eighteen-wheeler losing its brakes going downhill—not much can stop it. In other cases, milder risks may pile atop one another, with lots needed before the "point of no return." Perhaps this is the difference between children whose autism is visible seemingly from birth, and those whose autism shows up later, as a regression. There are many ways of accumulating these problems, leading to many ways of having autism.

By now you've seen, too, that at least in many cases there *is* a point of return, a chance to reverse the vicious circles and to create health-promoting circles instead. Or perhaps there are many points of return, many choices every single day that can help.

In this chapter, let's zoom out from your child to a bigger view—before your next child is born. Taking this perspective inevitably leads not just to your next child but also to you, your whole family, and the world we all share. I believe that when the science is in, we will see that people with autism are "canaries in the coal mine," the most susceptible, who are affected first by problems that may eventually reach us all.

One of my main research efforts right now is studying the younger siblings of children diagnosed with autism. My colleagues and I are looking at all sorts of brain and body indicators, from EEG and stress to metabolism, immune system, and toxic measures. Our goal is to test the idea that autism develops as a whole-body condition rather than being stamped from birth. We will not find out whether one treatment is better than another, but we will look at a wider array of brain and physical symptoms to see if there are signs of autism long before you can see the behaviors we now use for diagnosis. When our results and other studies now under way are completed, we should have a better early warning system for autism—and some benchmarks for studying prevention.

In the meantime, if you have any reason to think that your yet-to-be-born child is particularly vulnerable—because of genes, family history, dietary patterns, chemical or infectious exposures, or stress early in life—you may want to approach pregnancy with a particularly high level of vigilance and willingness to act. As Rose Blaire hopes, it might save a lot of heartache later.

I suggest following the "precautionary principle," or, in more common language: better safe than sorry. It's better to do a few, relatively simple things now to hopefully stop the downward cycle from picking up speed, than to have to cope with major health problems later. My advice, which basically involves adopting a healthier lifestyle, may help only your own well-being. The best case is that it will help your unborn child's, too.

Sources of Vulnerability

Not every child with autism has parents with health problems, but research shows that a surprising number of mothers, fathers, and other close relatives do have a history of ailments, including allergies, hormone problems, neurological, psychiatric, or gastrointestinal disorders, and chemical and/or environmental sensitivities. One study showed that parents diagnosed with schizophrenia, for example, had twice the risk of having a child with autism than parents without the diagnosis. The study, published in the prestigious journal *Pediatrics,* also found higher rates of depression and personality disorders among mothers, but not fathers. There may be a higher risk of cancer as well.

A small minority of people diagnosed with autism have a known genetic glitch, whether on the fragile X gene, idic(15), or the MeCP2 gene linked to Rett syndrome. This percentage may go up with further genetic research. Older parents are more likely to have children on the spectrum, particularly when there's a big age gap between the parents. This could mean that some kind of damage is occurring to the parents' egg or sperm, possibly from an environmental exposure. But as I hope I've convinced you by now, even with these known genetic glitches—as with PKU—there are many ways problems can show up, and potentially a range of strategies that will help.

The Blaires were completely surprised when Foster developed autism, as most families touched by the condition are. In retrospect, though, they see some things that might have been warning signs.

Rose had had immune problems nearly her entire life. She had regular bouts of arthritis and her tonsils were inflamed for years. As a child, her parents were opposed to taking them out, but she had been put on loads of antibiotics. She noticed that she had an annual pattern of getting sick—not when everyone else did in the winter, but during the spring and fall allergy seasons when grasses and molds would frequently bother her, suggesting that her allergies also wore down her immune system. Her white blood cell count was extremely high during her pregnancies with Foster and Nate, but her doctors didn't have her do anything about it.

In addition, Lewis recently learned that he has celiac disease, an immune problem that leaves him unable to safely digest gluten.

BEFORE AND DURING PREGNANCY

Pregnancy, birth, and early childhood are times of particular vulnerability, while the brain and digestive system develop and the body is exposed to the world for the first time.

We know surprisingly little about what's helpful and what's potentially dangerous to the fetus. Obviously, alcohol in excess and substance abuse can have a terrible impact on a child, and some medications are forbidden during pregnancy, but other than that, most mothers-to-be are just told to avoid cigarettes, eat healthy, not gain too much weight, and take prenatal vitamins.

The Blaires: Little Changes Made a Big Difference

When Rose did her Internet research about preventing autism in her third child, she didn't find much. But what she did find convinced her to change her diet, eating only organic and staying away from processed foods. She also avoided all pesticides, and harsh cleaners.

She had read that inflammation during pregnancy might be bad for the baby, so she added a vitamin B supplement and some fish oil and avoided getting a flu shot. She was glad she had finally had her tonsils out a few years before—they had been swollen most of her life, and were definitely inflamed during her previous two pregnancies.

"I made really little changes," she says—so little that they didn't do much to relieve her fear of having another child with autism. "I was so worried my entire pregnancy."

Rose got particularly anxious during every ultrasound when they measured her fetus's head. Large head size is a possible indicator of autism risk, and both Foster's and Nate's had been unusually large at birth.

Her pregnancy went smoothly, though, right up until the end.

She was two weeks past her due date when her labor kept starting and then stalling. She walked around in the hospital for about ten hours with her cervix stuck at 7 centimeters' dilation. Finally the doctor gave her a large dose of Pitocin—even though she'd asked him to keep the process slow and steady, because of her autism anxieties—and Jordan was delivered fifteen minutes later. Rose was furious, but Jordan was healthy and nearly three inches taller than both of his brothers had been, with a normal-sized head, although his face was bruised.

Jordan's early days went a long way toward easing Rose and Lewis's fears.

"Right away, he seemed more alert" than the other two had, Rose says. "He didn't cry as much. He had no problems with breastfeeding."

But Nate had been a happy baby, too. At first.

Food

As with other times of life, research indicates that it's prudent to maintain a high-nutrient-density, plant-based diet during pregnancy, with lots of multicolored vegetables and fruits, whole grains (if you can tolerate them), and high-quality proteins. Avoiding processed foods and food additives is also wise, because even if they were tested for safety in pregnancy, those tests are not designed to look for developmental issues like autism.

Mothers with nutrition problems often deliver babies with the same issues, so it's prudent to take a good prenatal vitamin. Nutrients that are believed to be particularly important during pregnancy are folic acid (to prevent certain birth defects), essential fatty acids, and vitamin D. For women not taking prenatal vitamins, a study showed a 60 percent higher risk of having a child with autism, with an even higher risk when mothers or infants had vulnerable genes related to methylation and folic acid.

One recent study showed that women who took 4,000 IU a day of vitamin D reduced their risk of preterm labor. Other nutrients to consider in order at least to avoid deficiency include zinc, cobalamin (vitamin B_{12}), and selenium—but research has not established appropriate levels for pregnant women, so it's important not to overdo these. Given methylation problems in autism, some methylated vitamins (e.g., methylcobalamin, also known as Methyl B_{12}) and methylated folate may prove more effective; but more studies need to be done as there could also be risks. It is best if you can get your vitamin and mineral levels (especially vitamin D) optimized before you get pregnant. Autism rates are particularly high among Somali populations in northern cities like Minneapolis and Toronto, and researchers are investigating whether that's because the mothers aren't getting enough sunshine to make adequate amounts of vitamin D. (Dark skin makes less vitamin D when exposed to the same amount of sunlight.)

There is data that a pregnant woman's immune response to infection may affect her fetus. We don't know whether allergic responses could have the same effect, but it is still probably a good idea to avoid foods and environmental triggers that cause you allergy problems. (I would be cautious about using any anti-allergy medications unless your doctor specifically directs you to use these and they have been safety tested in pregnancy.)

Toxins

Avoid as many environmental toxins as possible, particularly the ones you can control easily, such as alcohol, drugs, and pesticides. Try to use green household products, and stay away from mold.

Pregnancy is *not* the time to remodel your home. Opening up walls, refinishing floors, and doing virtually any other major repair project will kick up dust, release stuff that had been trapped in the walls, and introduce new chemicals into your environment, which means into your body and bloodstream—and potentially your baby—through your nose, lungs, mouth, gut, and skin. If you must remodel, stay in some other place during the work, and for long enough afterward that the dust has settled and the smell dissipated.

Pregnancy is not the time to remodel yourself, either. Your baby will love your nose just the way it is; elective surgery is just not a good idea right now.

Doing a detox program is a terrible idea during pregnancy or in the six to twelve months before becoming pregnant—it will release and circulate substances that could very well end up in your baby.

Avoid unnecessary medications and dental work. If you must take medicines, ask your doctor if they put you at risk for any nutrient deficiencies. Some antidepressants, for instance, deplete folate, and some seizure medications reduce carnitine—these are always important but especially so while you're pregnant. You may be able to help reduce the risk by supplementing with the nutrients, but talk to your doctor about it first.

Get the minimum number of ultrasounds. Avoid the temptation to take an extra peek, particularly if it's just to show your family and friends. Every medical procedure poses some risk, and it's best to avoid as many risks as possible right now.

Bugs

Infections during pregnancy can cause problems or, as I just mentioned, trigger an immune response that increases risk for neurodevelopmental conditions, including autism and schizophrenia. Research on this topic is not far enough advanced to specifically help with choosing preventive measures, but it's important to continue with your high-nutrient diet, stress reduction, and healthy sleep habits.

Step up your usual precautions for avoiding colds and other contagious bugs: Wash your hands often, particularly before you eat; don't share foods with others—including your incredibly cute older children; get a seasonal flu shot *before* getting pregnant, if possible. Reduce your risk of getting insect-borne illnesses by wearing long sleeves and pants and staying indoors at dusk, when mosquitoes are most active. Avoid eating raw animal products like sushi and shellfish (FoodSafety.gov has other tips on foods to avoid during pregnancy). Use a condom to protect against sexually transmitted diseases, particularly if your partner has had other recent sexual partners. And skip the trip to the tropics, particularly if you didn't grow up there, to keep risk of tropical diseases low.

Cats can transmit toxoplasmosis, an infection that can affect your unborn child's brain. During pregnancy get someone else to clean the cat box.

Stress

Stress during pregnancy is well known to affect development through immune and hormonal and other mechanisms. Stress can increase risk of infection, which you want to avoid.

As always, the best ways to reduce stress are to exercise regularly and get plenty of sleep. Take a gentle yoga class or an evening walk with your husband or push your older child in a stroller. Try to find childbirth classes that teach breathing and relaxation techniques, if you don't already know them.

AFTER YOUR BABY IS BORN

We don't have much research here, other than that exclusive breastfeeding is best for a child until solid food is introduced, and it's ideal to keep breastfeeding for at least the first year. Breastfeeding offers immune as well as nutritional support for your baby. A baby's immune system is very immature for the first few months of life; your breast milk will help keep him safe.

Breastfeeding will also encourage you to hold your child a lot, which is a great idea. Hold your infant as soon as you can after birth. If you bottle-feed or breastfeed, keep your baby's head propped up so the fluids don't pool in the back of the throat and go up the ear tubes, which can lead to ear infections.

There's some new research suggesting that the timing of when you introduce your child to solids, particularly foods with gluten, can make a big difference in the development of gluten sensitivities and celiac disease. This research is changing too much right now for me to make a reliable recommendation, but you may want to do some research or at least check with your doctor about the best age at which to introduce solids.

Your diet matters, too. Your child is getting proteins from you and can get sensitized or allergic to them. If your child seems uncomfortable or colicky, the first thing to consider is to stop them from eating potential allergens, such as gluten, dairy, eggs, peanut products, soy, seafood, and chicken, because these may be getting into your milk and bothering your baby. Again, a high-nutrient, plant-based diet is important. Also try to eat a varied diet and rotate your foods so you don't eat the same thing every day, since repeated exposure to the same foods can cause problems if you or your child has immune vulnerabilities.

In terms of supplements, there is research suggesting that cod liver oil or fish oil is beneficial. Consider a multivitamin for yourself, and extra vitamin D to get your levels up into the middle of the normal range.

Probiotics may also be helpful for maintaining a healthy balance of gut microbes, particularly if your child has been getting sick frequently. Some studies suggest that the children of mothers who take probiotics during pregnancy and breastfeeding are less likely to develop allergies, although this may depend on other things, too. Infant probiotics may help your child avoid colic and possibly avoid developing allergies as well. The risk of probiotics is low unless your child has severe immune problems.

Fish oil is important for you as a mom because essential fatty acids get depleted during pregnancy—you give much of your own supply to your baby to support their brain growth. Postpartum depression can be associated with essential fatty acid deficiency.

Infant vitamins can be very hit-or-miss, with some having just vitamin C, iron, and folate. Shop for a brand that gives you a wider spectrum of nutrients.

When you introduce solid foods, do it slowly, one food at a time, and look for reactions. If you see reactions, back off and see if they go away. If they do, then avoid that food for a while and look for alternatives. You may need help from a physician or dietitian. Of course, you should always get regular pediatric care for your baby. Try to find a pediatrician who is neither alarmist nor dismissive, but instead willing to listen— and respond—to your concerns about your child's autism risks.

However, at this point pediatricians are not advised to look at risks in early infancy. The official vigilance starts at eighteen months for the autism itself. Hopefully this will change in the next few years since a network of infant researchers has been producing data that may guide pediatricians as to what to look for and do much earlier.

The Blaires: Rough Beginnings

Foster Blaire had been a challenge from the start. Rose was seventeen years old when she gave birth to him, and she had to be induced and have Foster vacuumed out. As an infant, he had cried nonstop, and suffered from colic, ear infections, and skin rashes.

"From the beginning, we could tell there was something off," Rose says.

Foster learned a few words but lost them all at around fifteen months and has been nonverbal since. He showed obsessive behaviors at a young age, playing endlessly with his toy trains, spinning their wheels and lining them up, always in the same way. And he was racked by anxiety.

"This is normal. He's fine," Rose's pediatrician told her repeatedly. Once Foster was diagnosed, the pediatrician asked Rose for information about autism, admitting that he knew nothing except that autistic kids liked trains.

Nate seemed much different as a baby: happy, content, and never crying. But he developed a little eczema around seven or eight months, and though no one noticed it at the time, he began missing developmental milestones.

Rose had sought out a new pediatrician by then. This doctor, who was billed as having expertise in autism, said Nate was doing fine.

"Looking back now, we clearly see that Nate did have a delay. Even his pediatricians didn't pick up on it," Rose says.

Rose breastfed Nate until he was two and a half, since she hoped to save him from the seasonal allergies that had bothered her for years. (Still a teenager when Foster was born, Rose hadn't managed to breastfeed him at all, but she was determined to give Nate a better start in life.) Nate seemed to fall apart right after Rose stopped nursing. He began regressing, losing language, throwing constant tantrums. He stopped eating many foods.

Nate had his tonsils removed a year later to stop the nearly constant strep infections and antibiotic treatments. It seemed to help some. His language started coming back and he was on a faster track than his older brother. But he was still clearly on the autism spectrum.

During her third pregnancy, Rose vowed to find a pediatrician who would listen better to her concerns and provide her more guidance. She settled on an osteopathic pediatrician with a large practice in autism, and had her first visit during her thirty-fifth week of pregnancy.

When Jordan was born, Rose took him to the doctor right away because of the bruising on his face. He got an osteopathic treatment to help ease out the strains from being born. The bruises on his face cleared within twenty-four hours. Licensed physicians with osteopathic training use their hands to gently and softly ease the strains from the twists, turns, and pressures of the birth process.

"I was so worried he was going to develop jaundice like his brothers, and if it weren't for that treatment I bet he would have," she says. Jordan's osteopathic pediatrician says that her treatment improves blood flow and drainage so the body's natural circulation can take care of the bruising.

Then the doctor started Jordan on probiotics, and Rose on vitamin B_{12}. Rose breastfed exclusively and continued eating lots of fruits and vegetables and avoiding processed foods.

Hidden Allergies Uncovered

At three weeks old, Jordan had developed a respiratory infection and was breathing with those wheezy gasps that every parent dreads. Nate was having three or four allergy attacks a week, and Rose's seasonal allergies sometimes triggered asthma attacks, so she supposed Jordan had just inherited the family curse.

After Rose heeded her new doctor's advice, the changes astounded them all.

Jordan's lungs cleared up. He started sleeping longer at night and wasn't as gassy. He hasn't had any health problems in the year since.

Nate also tested positive for an egg allergy and deficiencies in zinc, iron, and vitamin B_{12}. Once he eliminated wheat and eggs and started taking supplements, he stopped having asthma attacks. Almost overnight, he went from three or four attacks a week to none at all.

He also started gaining ground in school. "He has a lot more language now; he can socially interact with others," Rose says. Nate's language was the level of a two-and-a-half-year-old before he changed his diet, and he hadn't been learning much. Now, a little over a year later, he's jumped up to the level of a five-year-old.

"It's amazing to see him doing really well now," Rose says. "He's really on his way."

Foster, the oldest, has also seen improvements, but not nearly as dramatic as his brothers'. He's not having regular stomachaches, diarrhea, or constipation, and his eczema has cleared up. He's grown six inches over the last year—now topping six feet one, perhaps because getting rid of wheat allowed his body to absorb more nutrients. But behaviorally he's no better, and he still has no language.

The pediatrician is getting ready to try another round of tests to see if there's anything more she can do to help Foster.

"In a really good mood, he's very pleasant to be around. He gets very excited," Rose says. "If he's not in a good mood, he's very loud, he won't look at you, he hides his face. Lately it's been up and down between the two."

Sometimes Foster has these moments of clarity, Rose says. "He'll say a word or look at you in a way that you think there's more going on than what he can express." A couple of years ago, for instance, Foster wanted a new pair of shoes. His parents refused. He already had eight pairs—why did he need a ninth? Then Foster made them watch a video he'd found on YouTube that says the first thing people notice about others is their shoes. He couldn't persuade them with his words, but he could use YouTube to find the perfect video to make his case. Rose and Lewis caved in the face of such logic and bought him the black slip-ons he wanted.

Rose has noticed changes in herself, too, from the diet. Her arthritis isn't bothering her anymore, and her allergies and asthma are much better. "I'm not as tired. I'm more energetic. I feel happier," she says. Getting rid of wheat has made Lewis feel much better, too.

Rose says it's a hassle not to be able to stop at fast-food restaurants anymore, or let the kids eat the pizza lunches at school, but it's definitely worth the inconvenience. The change was so simple, "yet makes a big difference."

Possible Signs of Trouble Brewing

Just as each of the Blaire boys showed early warning signs of trouble, so research is increasingly showing links between early life events and the later diagnosis of autism. These early problems don't necessarily mean a baby will develop autism, but it's prudent to aim for as much wellness and good function as possible.

Colic: Colic is something to be concerned about. Dr. Carine, from chapter 4, believes that a baby should be able to lie down after feeding and be comfortable. This is a "gray zone" issue—it is not a "disease" to have an uncomfortable child, but it could insidiously predispose toward problems later. A fussy baby is preoccupied with unpleasant bodily and sensory experiences, rather than openly taking in and exploring their environment. Many children diagnosed with autism were colicky as babies. We don't know for certain, but colic may be one of those signs that a vicious circle is beginning.

If your baby is formula-fed and has colic, consider changing formulas, but be cautious with soy formula since many infants and children are sensitive or allergic to soy. Consider discussing formula change with your pediatrician, including to hypoallergenic or elemental formula, if issues persist. (In elemental formula the proteins are all broken down to individual amino acids, which don't trigger allergies.)

Osteopaths such as Jordan's doctor say that infant colic can come from pressure on nerves governing digestion. A case of colic that does not respond to dietary or behavioral changes may get better with osteopathic treatments.

Gut problems: If your child develops chronic diarrhea or other stool or digestive problems, be very persistent in your efforts to get them better since this could cascade into a bigger set of problems. Get medical attention to look for reflux, allergies, infections, and other medical problems. Look hard for allergens in your own diet if you are breastfeeding, and try eliminating suspected foods. Also look at your child's formula and food, and try infant probiotics.

Large heads: Research is starting to suggest that large head size like Foster's can sometimes also be a warning sign for autism, though your pediatrician may not tell you that your child's head is unusually large. Rose remembers that she had a terrible time getting shirts over Foster's head. There is no treatment specifically for large heads, but addressing all the body and developmental problems, particularly allergies (many young children with severe allergies also have large heads), might help.

Eye contact and joint attention: Another early sign of autism is a lack of eye contact, or if a baby by nine months old still doesn't spontaneously look in the direction where someone is looking or pointing (this is called "joint attention"). Some of the newer early intervention programs designed with autism in mind more specifically target these skills. Perhaps there is a local infant intervention program that can help build your sensitivity and responsiveness to your child's cues.

Try using several senses at once in coordination. Use your words, face, and hands together to reinforce the message you are sending, which makes connections for your baby. Research shows that babies learn better when they get the same message through multiple sensory channels at once.

INFANT-PARENT SYNCHRONY

Your baby starts to learn to relate even before birth. He or she can be sensitive to the rhythms of mother's heartbeat and breathing, to her stress or happiness, and even to sounds, particularly mother's voice.

Immediately after birth, your baby starts learning how to relate to the world, and this is shaped by how people relate back. As the baby grows, she gains more ways to relate. Mother (and father, too) can get "in synch" with the baby, and the pair can act as a unit, sharing rhythms, each regulating the other, or both "coregulating" together.

Synchrony, or "coregulating," is a whole-body process, affecting everything from brain to hormones to stress response to immune system to digestion. It enriches and coordinates all the senses. It puts the family in a natural state of unconditional love. It can be as good as it gets.

Research shows differences in mother-infant synchrony in preterm as compared to term infants—the preterm babies have a harder time getting "in synch" spontaneously. It also shows that interventions aimed at enhancing this synchrony during the first year of life can have a significant impact on health, learning, and development. This connectedness between infants and parents lays the foundation for future relatedness.

In a baby with significant risk factors for autism, developing this connectedness may take extra effort, and you may need to learn more skills to get through to your baby and get the synchrony flowing.

Infections: Infections are part of life, but if they start happening a lot, think about immune, allergy, and nutrition issues, and toxic issues as well: Where is the vulnerability coming from? To protect your baby's gut bugs, try avoiding antibiotics if they are not absolutely necessary. Remember that antibiotics do nothing for viral infections like colds or flu; they only impact bacteria. And too many antibiotics can teach the bugs to develop resistance to treatment. The American Academy of Pediatrics does not recommend antibiotics at the beginning of ear or sinus infections, but rather only if a child starts to look seriously ill. There is some published data that osteopathic manipulative treatment may make ear infections milder or help avoid them, perhaps by helping drainage and preventing fluid buildup. If your child does need antibiotics, start him or her on probiotics and continue them for at least a month after the antibiotics are done. If you are breastfeeding and need antibiotics yourself, remember that your baby will get them, too, through your breast milk. In addition to taking antibiotics yourself, you may consider probiotics formulated for your infant.

Sucking and swallowing problems: Sucking and swallowing problems are an issue if they interfere with feeding, but they can also be a sign of problems that may interfere later on with speech and language. Swallowing air, which happens with a poor suck, can contribute to colic and to a cascade of problems that can lead to chronic GI issues. Inefficient swallowing may contribute to ear infections if milk goes up the ear canal to the middle ear.

Poor muscle tone and poor coordination of the mouth and tongue, as well as the shape of the mouth and throat, can cause these sucking and swallowing problems. Occupational therapy, a speech-language therapist specializing in suck and swallow difficulties, or cranial osteopathy may help. For low muscle tone problems cod liver oil and vitamin E in infant-appropriate doses may be helpful, research shows. If the low tone is more severe, talk to your pediatrician about getting an assessment for mitochondrial, metabolic, or genetic issues.

Vaccinations

Jordan received all his vaccines in a slightly spaced-out schedule to accommodate his early illness and his family history of immune problems.

He ran a mild fever after his DTaP (Diphtheria, tetanus, and pertussis) shot, but otherwise did fine.

We can't know whether getting wheat out of his mother's breast milk kept his immune system strong. But I think his pediatrician has it right: Do the things you *can* to help your child, so you can do the things you *must* do, like vaccinate.

Avoiding Toxins

We don't know precisely how all the chemicals in our everyday environment affect us, but there's plenty of research in animals—and now beginning in people—to suggest that some chemicals can mess with our hormones, including estrogen, which might increase cancer risk. Other chemicals have been linked to hyperactivity, developmental disorders, and organ damage. These chemicals can be found in regular household items such as canned food, plastic containers, fireproofed clothing and furniture, and cosmetics.

Here are some suggestions for minimizing your exposure to potentially dangerous chemicals:

- Wash your hands and your child's hands often. In addition to cutting down on germs, hand washing gets rid of dust, which may contain dangerous chemicals.
- Choose products that have fewer or no potentially dangerous chemicals. There are a number of online guides for this sort of thing, including www.goodguide.com.
- Stay away from pesticides in food and the air. See www .whatsonmyfood.org. Stay inside with the windows closed if authorities are spraying for mosquitoes, and try not to live too close to a farm where pesticides are used. The children of farmworkers are at much higher risk for a host of neurological and behavior problems, including autism, research shows.
- Minimize exposure to endocrine disrupters like plasticizers that make plastics moldable. See www.endocrinedisruption.org and http://e.hormone.tulane.edu. Making your own baby food can help with this. It's really not any harder to mash up a banana than to open a jar of banana baby food. Other foods can be pureed fairly

easily. A Vitamix or other strong blender or food processor can increase your options here.

- Don't microwave food in plastic. Glass is safer. Heat from microwaves and maybe the dishwasher can cause the chemicals to spread from the plastic into your food. Get rid of containers that have cracks, scratches, or white buildup.
- If you live alongside a major highway or in an industrial zone, consider moving if you can. Several studies have shown that children who live right near highways or power plants are at increased risk for autism. If you can't move, consider being extra careful with all the changes that you *can* make. You might also look into putting HEPA air filters in the rooms of your home.
- Favor natural materials over synthetic ones in your home, and choose low-toxic materials, paints, finishers, and cleaning products whenever possible. Petroleum-based products can emit gases that might be harmful over time.
- While an airtight house is good for energy efficiency, a house that doesn't let in a little fresh air also doesn't let toxins escape. Consider keeping some windows open at least a crack to make sure air circulates in and out.
- Protect your child from lead exposure. If you live in a pre-1980s house, make sure none of the old paint is exposed and chipping. Sometimes soil in urban yards and playgrounds can be tainted with lead. If you want to be an urban gardener, have your soil tested, or consider raised-bed gardens.
- If you still smoke, quit. Don't let people smoke in your house.

If You Suspect Problems

Early intervention programs may not specifically address autism but they do help with many of the delays that can precede an autism diagnosis. They may help slow down the cascade of complications. It is important to address these delays even if autism is not suspected, because all these problems put a drag on your child's development. To the extent you can minimize them, your child will have a better chance to learn and develop fully.

In the past few years research has clearly shown that early intervention can make a big difference in an autistic child's development. A study in the journal *Pediatrics* showed that the children in a program specifically targeting autism-related behaviors saw bigger increases in IQ, a faster pace of learning, and a reduction of their autism severity. Services in your area may not have caught up yet with this science, so it is not always easy to get a timely diagnosis of autism in a toddler. Insurance issues may complicate attempts to establish rapid-diagnosis programs and provide small children with support as early as possible. But it's still important to do the very best you can to get the services your child needs as soon as possible.

Rose, Cindy, and a number of the other parents I've introduced you to needed to advocate for themselves around this issue—insisting on a diagnosis, appropriate intervention, and adequate insurance coverage. Hopefully the process of diagnosis and early treatment will get easier with time, but I worry that as government budgets continue to shrink there will be less support for early intervention services and we will be slower to get more scientific research on effectiveness. This will put more burden on you.

The Blaires: Moving Forward

In the last three or four months, Rose has stopped worrying about Jordan's future. He's been talking, using sign language, and babbling. His face lights up when Rose or Lewis walks into the room.

Now that Jordan is getting older and the boys are all feeling better, they're starting to interact more, to build relationships with one another.

Nate is using some of his newfound language to talk for Foster, Rose says. "If I tell Foster to do something, he'll say [to Foster], 'Yes, you need to do this,'" she says. "He definitely tries to help Foster."

Foster doesn't seem to like the idea that his baby brother is growing up. "Don't stand up, don't stand up, don't stand up," Foster will repeat endlessly to Jordan. Though barely a toddler, Jordan seems to understand there's something different about Foster. When he wants to talk to his big brother, he'll tap him on the shoulder first, Rose says—sensing, it seems, that he needs to get Foster's attention in a different way than everyone else's.

Foster is also protective of the baby, getting upset if strangers come near the little boy who looks so much like his dad and middle brother. When it's time to say good night, Foster will sign or wave good night to Jordan—and only Jordan.

"Having Jordan is the best thing that could have happened to us," Rose says. He's a joy to have in the house, and without him they wouldn't have discovered everyone's dietary problems.

Rose's only regret is that she didn't give up wheat earlier. If she had, she's convinced, Nate at least wouldn't have developed autism. We'll never know what would have happened. Or what will yet. Jordan might still develop autism, or he might not have regardless of his parents' and doctor's efforts. Nate might catch up developmentally, or he might not. The Blaires might figure out another way to help Foster.

For now, though, Rose and Lewis are happy with the present and starting to look optimistically toward the future.

"If Jordan continues to do really well, we might discuss having another child," Rose says. "It would be nice . . . We always wanted to have a large family."

A Healthier World

In this book I've focused on things you can do for your child, and in this chapter I've shown that this can apply to yourself, your next baby, and your whole family.

Are there things we can do as a society to reduce risk and increase health? I think so.

I am sure others have already told you about health risks from junk food, food additives, and household products. Now that you are aware of these things, it may seem like lots of extra work to make healthy choices.

Imagine if all your food choices were healthy. Imagine if all your products were safe. How much effort would we save? How much better would our quality of life be? How many fewer people would be sick?

As I see it, the suffering of autism and of many other chronic illnesses is tied together with the problems on our planet. Our modern way of life exploded on us before we knew how risky some of our progress could be.

Could the solutions all be related, too? Could making our food supply healthier and our products safer reduce risk for everyone? I think so.

Around the United States and the world, people are setting up centers for those with autism in rural areas or on organic farms, where working with plants and animals is part of the therapy—like the Center for Discovery in central New York state. These could be seeds of something much bigger.

Just as you need to learn to read your child's signals, we need to learn, or relearn, how to have a healthy relationship with the earth, how to be sensitive and responsive to the signals it is sending us.

The United Nations released a report in 2011 saying that we could double the world's food supply in ten years if we changed over to "agro-ecology"—organic farming. We could also restore jobs and reduce poverty around the world. The report concluded that the heavy use of chemical fertilizers, pesticides, and petroleum in conventional agriculture is not efficient, not economically feasible, is hard on our planet, is depleting our soils, and is making us sick.

Meanwhile, the food we get from this process is adding to our own risk: too many chemicals, not enough nutrients. Some people even describe the plant foods we get from these conventional farms as "inflamed" themselves due to far too few minerals in the soil. How can we heal ourselves when even our food is sick?

As you work to build the health of your child, yourself, and your family, you are voting with your feet and your pocketbook for better health options for everyone.

And as you move forward, you will find new friends and new communities who will help you and give you support and whom you will help as well.

Many are already finding that the Autism Revolution is about much more than autism. Anyone can join this revolution.

I wish you the best on your journey forward.

ACKNOWLEDGMENTS

No book is ever the work of one or two people. The communities of people who have influenced the development of this book are vast, and we could not ever begin to list everyone to whom we owe our deep gratitude. Here we would like to acknowledge the inspiration we received from our friends who have autism or whose families are touched by it; the scientists, doctors, and scholars who helped us refine the ideas in this book; and the rich tapestry of often vital contributions from others who provided moral, editing, and/or technical support during the eighteen months it took us to write it. That list includes: Anat Baniel, Judith Bluestone (deceased), Ali Carine, the Autism Society, Ted Carr (deceased), Abha and Ved Chauhan, Marnie Cochran, Marguerite Colston, Robyn Cosford, Olav Albert Christophersen, Georgia Davis, Geri Dawson, Judy Endow, Jill Escher, Deborah Fein, Donna Ferullo, Carey Goldberg, Matthew Goodwin, June Groden, Lee Grossman, Stephan Hagopian, Susan Hahn, Peter Hahn, Owen and Sarah Hahn, Patrick Hanaway, Todd Helmus, Robert Hendren, Elizabeth Horn, Ginger Houston-Ludlum, Mark Hyman, Linda Konner, Laurette Janak, Bryan Jepson, Roy John (deceased), Jane Johnson, Tal Kenet, Marcel Kinsbourne, Charles Krebs, Michael Kuchta, Joel Lefever, Ilyse Levine Kanji, Priyanka Krishnan, Richard Levins, Michael Lerner, Richard Lord, Robert Ludwig, Alison MacNeil, Paul Mankiewicz, Katherine Martien, John Martin, Woody McGinnis, David McKee, Meenakshi Mal, Michael Merzenich, Jane Moncreiff, Laurent Mottron, Brenda Smith Myles, Shelia Opperman, Craig Pangburn, Rosalind Picard, Tom Pitoniak, John Reed, Glenn Rothfeld, Sarah Stockwell, Georges St. Laurent, Cliff Saron, Judith and John Schmitz, Trent Schroyer, George Scailabba, Maya Shetreat-

Klein, Julie Silver, Stephen Smith Jim Smyth, Natalie Ramm, Marie Taft, Theoharis Theoharides, Transcend Research Program Staff, Juliet Ucelli, Gianfranco Valent, Judy van de Water, Hanne Bjørg Walker, Amy Wetherby, Martha Welch, Harriet and Ronald Weintraub, Mark Westaway, Janet Wygal, and Rachel Zimmerman.

APPENDIX A

Ten Tips for Helping People with Autism

1. **Go for the extraordinary.** You may feel that you know your child is "in there" somewhere. Trust your feeling. See your child's hidden gifts, even if they are blocked by lots of confusion and difficulties. Don't define your child by his or her problems—they grew out of a cascade of challenges that you can address together slowly, carefully, and deliberately. Don't aim for "normal." People with autism are capable of astounding insights and creativity. Your goal should be to rejoice in their strengths and shore up their vulnerable spots, not to "fix" them.

2. **Know what you can't control—and what you can.** The set of genes we are born with is what we will have for life, but that doesn't mean our future is foretold. The power of individual genes is shaped by our environment. Your aim should be to create as supportive and nourishing an environment as possible—for yourself as well as your loved one with autism.

3. **Repair and support cells and cycles.** Everything we do relies on our cells. How well we do it all is affected by our cellular health. Problems in cells create slowdowns and glitches; nourishing them well will make them more energetic and efficient. This solid foundation for your child's whole body and brain is well worth your serious effort.

4. **Get gut and immune systems on your side.** Napoleon Bonaparte once said that an "army marches on its stomach," meaning that a fighting force will only be strong if it is well fed. Our digestive system gives us energy and building materials, and our immune system relies on the gut and its vast array of gut bugs to learn what's friendly and fight what's dangerous. Our digestive and immune systems are vulnerable to problems because they are exposed to the outside world. But that also means they are accessible to our efforts to fortify them—and when we help them, we help the whole body.

5. **Build better brain health.** Our brains need energy and nutrition supplies. The neurons you have for life depend on partnerships with a good blood supply and networks of other brain cells, which grow and change and respond to the environment. You can build brain health by reducing blockages like those caused by inflammation, and by feeding brain cells the nutrients they need to function. Better brain health will help restore the brain's full powers.

6. **Calm brain chaos.** Remember the last time you went to a busy department store or museum, a state fair or an amusement park. You were probably exhausted when you got home, worn-out not just from the activities you did, but from the stress of all that chaos. The brains of people with autism can create that level of bedlam and worse all the time. Sensory, sleep, seizure, speech and language, and other brain-based issues increase your child's stress. Understanding how your child's brain makes them feel, and having concrete steps you can take to help with this, will make their world (and yours) more manageable.

7. **Join your child's world.** Look for the hidden reasons behind what your child does, especially when it is hardest to imagine any. Challenging or bizarre behavior is usually a signal that something is not right, either outside or inside their bodies. Learn to decode your child's messages, and communicate in ways he or she can understand. Take it as slowly as necessary. Without judgment, teach them step by step the simple things that come naturally to people without autism. If you deeply join their world and love them unconditionally just as they are, they will feel safer and will blossom more easily.

8. **Love, rejoice, and make breakthroughs.** Once you get in synch with your child's world, find ways to gently broaden it. Enrich their experience. Give them physical activities they might not choose on their own so they can feel how their bodies move in space. Help them channel their special interests into skills. Build bridges between your way of experiencing and theirs. Help them expand their comfort zone and means of communicating. Give them room to find their own inner rhythms and feelings. Then step back, let their creativity flow, and celebrate.

9. **Lead the revolution!** There's a ridiculous amount expected of you as the parent of a child with autism. In addition to just making it through the day, you need to carefully track your child's progress to see what's working and what

isn't worth the effort. Share what you learn and it may help others, too. Advocate for research that gives us a handle on how to support your child the most. You can help us all take a revolutionary fresh look at autism so we can address our own as well as society's autism problem. Let's all be part of the solution.

10. **Do it for yourself, your next baby, your family, and your world.** Learn to look at autism as something that develops, not something that is destined. Viewing autism as the outcome of a cascade of events gives you strategies for slowing or stopping that cascade—or even dialing it back. Your autism challenge can give you the impetus to strongly support the health of your whole family, your future children, and your environment.

APPENDIX B

Sample Forms for
Tracking Your Data

	Wake-up	Earlier morning	Later morning	Noon	Earlier afternoon	Later afternoon	Dinner	Earlier evening	Later evening	Middle of night
Events										
Attention, Focus or Distracted (Scale: 1 = very focused, 10 = extreme discontrol)										
Food, Drinks										
Meds & Supplements										
Gut, Bathroom										
Toxins—Exposed, Avoided, Reactions										
Bugs and Allergens—Exposures, Reactions										
Stress, Seizures, Sleep										
Behavior, Mood, Anxiety, Calm										
Stimming, Tics										
Sensory Breaks, Exercise										
Mind-Body Activities (Yoga, relaxation, breathing, animals, gardening)										
Creativity, Humor, Jokes										
Speech, Language, Echolalia, Other Communication										

Log extra details in margins or on back of sheet

DAILY FOOD LOG

DATE: _____

TYPE OF FOOD	Morning	Midday	Afternoon	Evening	Night
Vegetables					
Fruits					
Meat or Poultry					
Fish					
Beans					
Dairy (milk, cheese, cream)					
Yogurt, Kefir					
Cultured Vegetables					
Pizza					
Bread					
Cake, Cookies					
Pasta					
Candy					
Soda					
Enter more foods					

DAILY FOOD LOG (continued)

DATE: _____

TYPE OF FOOD	Morning	Midday	Afternoon	Evening	Night
How Food Was Prepared					
Raw					
Cooked					
Fresh					
Fried					
From Box or Package					
Colors					
Red					
Orange					
Yellow					
Green					
Blue or Purple					
Black					
Brown					
Beige					
White					
Foods Not Tolerated					
Food Reactions					

DAILY TREATMENT OR INTERVENTION LOG (Meds, Supplements, Therapies, etc.)

DATE:

TREATMENT OR INTERVENTION	Dose or Time Duration	Morning	Midday	Afternoon	Evening	Night	Comment

ONGOING TREATMENT/INTERVENTION START/CHANGE/STOP LOG

TREATMENT OR INTERVENTION	Date Begun or Stopped	Dose or How Often	Why Started or Stopped	What help or transformations are you hoping for? What is still left for you to do?

APPENDIX C

Whole-Body Systems Summary

Here are the main points I make in this book, summarized from a systems perspective. I talk about how autism is composed of many levels, that they are all interconnected in a web, and that you can make progress by helping lots of the parts of the web. The goal is to help your child be everything they can be, to let their full capabilities flower. This approach is rooted in systems thinking and in the recent explosion of systems biology. Here I make those connections more explicit for you.

1. The idea that autism is a fixed state of impairment is not proven but is an assumption. Moreover, this assumption can keep you from recognizing many practical ways to help your child. You have a choice about how you think and what assumptions you use to guide your actions. Here are some basic things to remember:

    a. Autism is not intrinsically an impairment or mental deficiency. It is sometimes associated with impairment, but it is not defined by impairment. In fact many people with autism are remarkably gifted.

    b. Many parts of autism are changeable, not permanent, hardwired, or set in stone.

    c. Problems that look like permanent "impairments" in many cases can be due to blockages or to poor coordination of your child's resources. This blockage or poor coordination may be chronic, so chronic that it looks permanent. Their capabilities may be "offline." Yet your child may be fully capable once the roadblocks are removed or the coordination improved.

d. Therefore, while your child needs to learn and build skills, they also need to get unnecessary blockages out of the way.

2. Obstruction or weak coordination can come from genes or environment or both together. When you have a strong genetic influence, you need only weak environmental triggers. With strong environmental triggers, you may not need much genetic influence.

a. Genes, gene expression, and gene damage are all ways genes can contribute. You can't change the first but you can make choices about things that affect the second and third.

b. Food, toxins, bugs, and stress are major classes of environmental inputs that physically and mentally affect us. We can make small changes or big changes, but even small changes can sometimes have large effects.

c. Your child also needs to learn new things and perceive and categorize differences in the world. The most general term for this is getting *information*. Gregory Bateson, one of the great systems thinkers of the twentieth century (with whom I studied) said that "information is a difference that makes a difference." When you teach your child or when your child has sensory experiences (that is, all the time) they need to be able to handle the information. That's how they make sense of the world. That's how "input" turns into "information" or "news you can use." If the information is given in ways their system can't handle, they can't organize it and make distinctions with the information. Instead it can contribute to overloading them and can lead to dysfunction.

d. All levels of our experience, from molecules to cells to our guts digesting food, to our immune system figuring out how to deal with new things, to our brains processing new input—all involve handling new information.

i. Every level of our whole-body system needs information in ways it can handle.

ii. Every level of our whole-body system can get in trouble if its inputs come in forms it can't handle.

3. Autism's problems occur at all levels, including genes, cells, organs, systems, brain, sensation, movement, emotion, behavior, and learning. We don't know enough to say where the problems start, and I think they probably start differently in different people. But it does appear that once a vulnerable system begins to get disrupted, the disruption spreads through many other levels.

a. Given poor-quality inputs from food, toxins, bugs, and stress the system can get a lot of "encouragement" to move to greater degrees of disruption.

b. Your child's whole-body system may already be so overloaded that it has less bandwidth for handling information that arrives in hard-to-digest forms. This includes too much noise, allergens in food, toxic exposures, infections, and much more. But the world is full of sources of overload. As a result your child gets lots of pushes toward disruption of functioning, not just behaviorally but at every level of their system.

c. Regression into autism that some children experience may be what occurs when the disruption hits a tipping point and causes a state shift, which may occur suddenly or more gradually. *State shift* means a transformation of the system so it functions differently—in this case with lots of hangups it may not have had before. This state shift is likely to affect many levels at the same time. For those children who do not obviously regress, they could have undergone a process like this while they were developing in the womb, before they were born.

d. What you see as behavior or cognitive problems may be downstream of underlying problems at deeper levels (as with cells, systems, sensory thresholding) that you can't see. Without suspecting a contribution from these underlying levels you may tend to interpret what you see as primarily psychological or motivation based. Parents can even take it personally and feel like their child is being deliberately oppositional or manipulative. When you feel this way, imagine you are wearing zoom lenses that can peer deeply into the inner world of your child, from their feelings to their body experience all the way down to their cells and molecules. Imagine that your child is experiencing disorganization and even discomfort at many or all of these levels. The "bad" or "disruptive" behaviors or the "impairments" you see without those zoom lenses are actually the product of all the disruption at all of your child's hidden levels.

4. Progressive dysfunction is therefore a result of system overload. If we define *stress* as what happens when demands exceed available resources, your child is experiencing stress at many or all levels of their system.

a. Once the system starts to be in a disrupted configuration, more overload reinforces the problems and makes them worse.

b. The more the system is stressed, the less information it can handle. What might once have been "signal" starts to be "noise"—that is, chaos that may not contribute to organization and development but may instead lead to stress, fear, meltdowns, and withdrawal, as well as lots of body problems as your child's cells and organs and brain get overwhelmed. (In information theory and engineering this is called reducing or degrading the "signal-to-noise ratio.")

c. In order to overcome this situation you need to reduce the noise, so the system can start perceiving signal again.

      d.   Reducing the "noise" is not just a sensory issue. It means reducing as much as possible the disruptive signals going to all levels of the system, from your child's cells to their organs to their brain and nervous system.

      e.   At the same time you need to give your child's system what it needs and can handle. This means sound that is not too loud but just right, instructions your child can follow, tasks that your child can succeed at, foods full of the nutrients your child's body needs to do its work and get better, and lots of rest, comfort, and love.

5. Progressive dysfunction at every level of the system occurs in shades of gray, not black and white, not either you have it or you don't. It's a spectrum of spectrums, because there are shades of gray at all the various levels.

      a.   This has made it hard for medicine to handle autism—because its symptoms are i) all over the place, and ii) not necessarily consistent with or severe enough to meet criteria for definitions for existing disease categories.

      b.   Science is moving toward shades of gray at the cellular level. It used to be that cells were either healthy or entering a cell-death process. Emerging now is a sense that the cells can be in effect "chronically ill" or dysfunctional without being dead. This means that they can in principle bounce back.

      c.   Many of the brain problems being identified both in autism and in other conditions are also in shades of gray, not black and white, and research and clinical experience are starting to show that they can be shifted toward a more functional direction.

      d.   Thinking in terms of shades of gray allows you to gently nudge your child's health and learning along at every moment of the day and at every level. These little moment-by-moment advances may add up to big system changes over time.

6. What I am offering you is a way of looking at your child's issues so that you find opportunities to remove stress and add resources. This will help your child's system to reorganize in healthier ways, freeing your child to use more of their capabilities. This approach makes sense even if your child has serious problems like genetic abnormalities or other serious illnesses.

      a.   If this is started early enough (for example, before conception, during pregnancy, or very early in life) it may be a program for prevention.

      b.   What I wish for your child is for them to be able to use everything they have, to have lots of choices and options about what they do and how they respond to the world. This doesn't mean being average, but being comfortable, being everything they can be, coming into their full flowering, which will make them extraordinary.

7. System resources can be improved in many ways.

      a.   Based on luck but also on choices you can control, you can move things in two directions:

      i.   Food, toxins, bugs, and stress can add to your child's systems overload by piling more challenges on top of the genetic vulnerability and prior environmental disruptions they already have.

      ii. Thoughtful, healthy handling of food, toxins, bugs, and stress can also decrease overload by reducing problem exposures and adding to the system's resources. This will give your child's whole-body system the best chance of regenerating health and richly integrated function.

  b. Exposing your child to new information through teaching and helping them build new skills can also increase your child's system's resources if you offer these experiences in ways your child can perceive and integrate.

  c. Nothing is too small. Even little choices can have leverage. They can make a lot of difference in a delicately balanced, struggling system.

8. Much of what I am saying has parallels in a lot of other chronic and neurodevelopmental conditions, such as ADHD, learning disabilities, asthma, diabetes, obesity, and even Alzheimer's, cancer, and many more. Common genes and common environmental stressors are being found across all these conditions. Thus we can learn from progress in other conditions. And people with these other problems can learn from your successes with autism.

  a. We don't know why common genetic and environmental vulnerabilities lead to different diseases. Maybe it is a combination of timing in development, specifics of genetic vulnerability, and specific features (such as chemistry) of the environmental overloads.

  b. While there may be some interventions that specifically and uniquely target autism, I think it is plausible to expect that to a large degree we will make gains from interventions that are more generic rather than autism-specific.

9. Intervening or treating at just one level may help a lot. But your child may still be left with many residual issues, at medical, behavioral, learning, or emotional levels. I think an intensive effort at multiple levels gives your child a better chance of turning things around.

  a. Targeting one thing at a time may leave your child's system vulnerable to returning to the problems it is familiar with because the inertia at all the other levels pushes it back.

  b. Targeting multiple levels at once can help leave behind that dysfunctional state or "set point" and give your child more resources to shift into a healthier state. This healthier state can become more stable over time as you persist.

  c. Therefore, for best results I recommend removing burdens and adding resources at every level where it is possible to do so without causing undue risk. This will take stress off the system at lots of levels and give the maximum chance for self-correction and resiliency. The best foundation for doing this is to do the best you possibly can through addressing food, toxins, bugs, and stress.

d. Even if more aggressive treatments are needed, such as heavy-duty pharmaceutical interventions, you should cover all the basic levels first or in parallel, to minimize the need for these more side effect–laden approaches and maximize your child's chances to do well. This means doing the best possible job with foods, toxins, bugs, and stress.

10. Many of the things that can help are everyday interventions, like food and product choices, and ways of communicating with your child. Many may work for your child when they are ready but not before that, some may be outgrown, and some never make sense.

a. Taking a coordinated approach to the many levels of your child's issues is a way of dealing with autism that can be very hard to test with standard clinical trial testing methods, which are best at testing one thing at a time. Therefore, my goal is to help inform your judgment in looking for interventions that are safe and make sense in their biology, their psychology, and their information content, even if they haven't been proven beyond a shadow of a doubt either singly or in the combinations you are using.

b. Emerging data-gathering methods such as Web-based patient and family databases may add group knowledge about these everyday things in ways that were never before possible.

c. As you and others in your situation get more control of the situation and experience successes, you may have more bandwidth for helping the world to undergo a state shift so that it has more things in it that promote health and less things that promote vulnerability.

d. You and your experiences can have a lot to teach and offer the world.

APPENDIX D

Ten Tips for Doctors, Therapists, and Scientists

Here are some things doctors, therapists, and scientists can do, individually and in groups, to spur on the Autism Revolution and the people who need it the most.

1. **Meet, listen to, and learn** from people with autism and their families and caregivers. You can start by watching videos of people with autism and what they have to say and show. (I am including some links in the resource section.) But real face-to-face time is incredibly valuable. Listen to family members, to experienced skilled teachers and therapists, to people with in-depth, daily, long-term experience. Learn what it is like every day.
2. **Think about the whole person.** You as a scientist or clinician may want to treat "core" features of autism. But in the everyday lives of people with autism and their families some of the things that are most disruptive are the sleep problems, the GI problems, and the seizures. Remember the words of Sir William Osler: "The good physician treats the disease; the great physician treats the patient who has the disease."
3. **Be open** to surprises and observations really different from what you've been taught. If a child does better with fever or steroids or loses their diagnosis, maybe it's telling you something new about autism, not proving they didn't have autism in the first place. You may also learn about potential for scientific

research by listening carefully to parents, who know their children better than anyone. This is how the fever study I discussed in chapter 5 was designed and performed—clinicians took seriously what parents had been telling them. We still don't know how close to the core of autism this discovery of the fever effect may be. But it totally violates what professionals and the public had been taught to believe about autism. And it promises to be a gold mine for new insights.

4. **Look beyond blanket diagnoses** and work on viewing each of your patients, research subjects, or study questions as a giant web with many threads. Look for ways to help or take account of any accessible parts of the web.

5. **Take problems seriously** before they get really serious. Probe for "gray zone" issues, which may be relatively easy to treat, before they reach a level of severity that makes them harder to resolve.

6. **Think physiologically.** Think about how systems work in the body. Your patients may have some idiosyncratic problems (like unusual chemical or infectious exposures or metabolic, immune, or genetic glitches) or combinations of problems that lead them to deviate from the textbooks. But you can still use physiology to reason about how to help. Read Denis Noble's marvelous book *The Music of Life* to hear the author's perspective on how physiology rather than genes is where the action is in living systems.

7. **Become fascinated with the environment,** what we know and don't know, and how food, toxins, bugs, and stress impact our biology. This may be painful but it's hugely enlightening. Learn about environmentally vulnerable physiology and how to support and protect it.

8. **Learn about systems biology.** Our technologies and our knowledge are way ahead of our medical, testing, and regulatory practices. They're also way ahead of what most clinicians have time or resources to do. Systems biology thinking can also be hard to incorporate into research because many peer reviewers still think in older reductionist terms. But it's also a habit of mind that you can adopt even as a beginner. This way of thinking about interactions and context will make you more humble but also help you tune in better to many more ways you can be of service.

9. **Explore practical approaches** to systems biology that are emerging in medicine. One of them is *P4 medicine:* Predictive, Personalized, Preventive, and Participatory, from the Institute for Systems Biology, which is developing partnerships with major academic centers such as Ohio State University. This approach has attracted a lot of brilliant people. It gives us a sense of what will become possible when science advances to allow more systematic testing, although for now they mainly focus on the predictive power of genes and on addressing adult problems.

Another approach is *functional medicine,* which defines itself as a science-based approach to dealing with primary prevention and underlying causes rather than focusing on symptoms. One of its main tenets is that health is not just the absence of disease but rather a positive vitality—in effect "making life all it can be." I think that functional medicine works to strike a balance among genes, environment, metabolism, immunology, structure, and other aspects of whole-body, whole-systems medicine. All of these levels are needed to address the complexities of autism—and many other chronic illnesses. The part of functional medicine that I find most valuable is how it provides a framework for organizing your approach to patients and problems. You can use this organizing framework now, even while you build your knowledge base and even while the science is still accumulating. It can help you to be systematic in how you work to lower the overall burden across each person's own complex web, and to build supports. Certification and advanced practice modules are available for licensed healthcare providers through the Institute for Functional Medicine, www.functionalmedicine.org. I am also including several functional medicine textbooks and articles under Further Reading.

10. **Take time to remember** why you chose your profession in the first place at the level of your core values and aspirations. Think about how you can ground yourself in that vision to be as resourceful as you can for each patient, each study, everything you do. Get a sense of how that connects you with systems thinking and taking account of the whole web.

APPENDIX E

Further Reading

GUIDES FOR PARENTS

R. Dietert and J. Dietert, *Strategies for Protecting Your Child's Immune System: Tools for Parents and Parents-to-Be.* Singapore: World Scientific, 2010.

P. Kluth, *You're Going to Love This Kid.* Baltimore: Paul H. Brookes, 2003.

E. Notbohm. *Ten Things Every Child with Autism Wishes You Knew.* Arlington, TX: Future Horizons, 2005.

R. Sears, *The Autism Book: What Every Parent Needs to Know About Early Detection, Treatment, Recovery and Prevention.* Sears Parenting Library. New York: Little, Brown, 2010.

K. Seroussi and L. Lewis, *The Encyclopedia of Dietary Interventions for the Treatment of Autism and Related Disorders.* Pennington, NJ: Sarpsborg Press, 2008.

S. Shore, L. G. Rastelli, and T. Grandin, *Understanding Autism for Dummies.* Hoboken, NJ: For Dummies, 2006.

R. Smith and B. Lourie, *Slow Death by Rubber Duck: The Secret Danger of Everyday Things.* Berkeley, CA: Counterpoint, 2010.

F. R. Volkmar and L. A. Wiesner, *A Practical Guide to Autism: What Every Parent, Family Member, and Teacher Needs to Know.* Hoboken, NJ: Wiley, 2009.

N. Wiseman, *Could It Be Autism?* New York: Crown Archetype, 2006.

———, *The First Year: Autism Spectrum Disorders: An Essential Guide for the Newly Diagnosed Child.* New York: Da Capo Lifelong Books, 2009, and www .firstsigns.org.

PERSONAL PERSPECTIVES ON AUTISM

Judy Endow, *Paper Words: Discovering and Living with My Autism*. Shawnee Mission, KS: Autism Asperger Publishing, 2009.

Temple Grandin, *Thinking in Pictures: My Life with Autism*. Expanded ed. New York: Vintage, 2010.

————, *The Way I See It: A Personal Look at Autism and Asperger's*. 2nd ed. Arlington, TX: Future Horizons, 2011.

Portia Iversen, *Strange Son*. New York: Riverhead, 2006.

Tito Rajarshi Mukhopadhyay, *How Can I Talk If My Lips Don't Move? Inside My Autistic Mind*. New York: Arcade, 2011.

————, *The Mind Tree*. New York: Arcade, 2011.

Dawn Prince-Hughes, *Songs of the Gorilla Nation: My Journey Through Autism*. New York: Three Rivers Press, 2005.

John Elder Robison, *Be Different*. New York: Crown Archetype, 2011.

————, *Look Me in the Eye: My Life with Asperger's*. New York: Broadway, 2008.

Ralph James Savarese, *Reasonable People: A Memoir of Autism and Adoption: On the Meaning of Family and the Politics of Neurological Difference*. New York: Other Press, 2007.

HEFTIER READING

D. Amaral, G. Dawson, D. Geschwind, eds., *Autism Spectrum Disorders*. Oxford: Oxford University Press, 2011.

J. Bland et al., *Clinical Nutrition: A Functional Approach*. 2nd ed. Gig Harbor, WA: Institute for Functional Medicine, 2004.

A. Bralley and R. Lord, *Laboratory Evaluations for Integrative and Functional Medicine*. 2nd ed. Duluth, GA: Metametrix Institute, 2008.

A. Chauhan, V. Chauhan, and T. Brown, eds., *Autism: Oxidative Stress, Inflammation, and Immune Abnormalities*. Boca Raton, FL: Taylor & Francis/CRC Press, 2009.

K. Fitzgerald and J. Bralley, *Case Studies in Integrative and Functional Medicine*. Duluth, GA: Metametrix Institute, 2011.

D. Jones, L. Hoffman, and S. Quinn, *21st Century Medicine: A New Model for Medical Education and Practice*, available free online. www.functionalmedicine.org/content_management/files/21stCentMed-FullDocument.pdf

S. Knox, "From 'omics' to complex disease: a systems biology approach to gene-environment interactions in cancer. *Cancer Cell International*, 2010, 10: p. 11. www.cancerci.com/content/10/1/11.

B. Levin, *Environmental Nutrition*. Vashon Island, WA: HingePin Press, 1999.

The Textbook of Functional Medicine. 2nd ed. Gig Harbor, WA: Institute for Functional Medicine, 2008.

A. Zimmerman, ed. *Autism: Current Theories and Evidence*. Totowa, NJ: Humana Press, 2008.

SOME AUTISM RESOURCES AND ORGANIZATIONS

American Academy of Pediatrics: www.aap.org/healthtopics/autism.cfm.

Autism Research Institute: www.autism.com.

Autism Society: www.autism-society.org.

Autism Speaks: www.autismspeaks.org.

Autism Treatment Network: www.autismspeaks.org/science/programs/atn/.

National Database for Autism Research: ndar.nih.gov.

U.S. Centers for Disease Control and Prevention: www.cdc.gov/ncbddd/autism/index.html.

TREATMENT-TRACKING DATABASES AND RESOURCES FOR PARENTS

Autism 360: www.autism360.org.

ChARM: www.charmtracker.com.

Patients Like Me: www.patientslikeme.com.

Self-tracking data resources: www.quantifiedself.com

GENERAL INFORMATION

A. M. Wetherby and N. Wiseman, Autism Video Glossary: http://www.autismspeaks.org/video/glossary.php.

Autism Internet Modules: www.autisminternetmodules.org.

BIOMEDICAL AND ENVIRONMENTAL INFORMATION

www.autismbiomed.com

www.autismbiorefs.info

www.autism.com/pro_biomedical_research.asp#Biomedical

www.autismwhyandhow.org

www.endocrinedisruption.com/endocrine.TEDXList.overview.php

www.endocrinedisruption.org

www.e.hormone.tulane.edu

www.healthandenvironment.org/cgi-bin/portal.cgi

www.epa.gov/epahome/commsearch.htm

BOOK AND AUTHOR WEBSITES

www.TheAutismRevolution.org

www.MarthaHerbert.org

www.KarenWeintraub.com

NOTES

CHAPTER 1. GO FOR THE EXTRAORDINARY

6   *Studies of home videos and direct observations:* Werner and Dawson, "Validation of the phenomenon of autistic regression using home videotapes," *Archives of General Psychiatry,* 2005, 62: pp. 889–95.

6   *In 2008 I was among a group of researchers:* Helt et al., "Can children with autism recover? If so, how?" *Neuropsychology Review,* 2008, 18: pp. 339–66.

7   *When I first got involved in autism research:* Croen et al., "The changing prevalence of autism in California," *Journal of Autism and Developmental Disorders,* 2002, 32: pp. 207–15.

7   *As I write, the figure is approaching 1 in 100:* Kogan et al., "Prevalence of parent-reported diagnosis of autism spectrum disorder among children in the US, 2007," *Pediatrics,* 2009, pp. 1395–1403.

7   *Autism involves the whole body:* Herbert, "Autism: A brain disorder or a disorder that affects the brain?" *Clinical Neuropsychiatry,* 2005, 2: pp. 354–79, www.marthaherbert.org/library/Herbert-autismbrainoraffectingbrain.pdf; Coury, "Medical treatment of autism spectrum disorders," *Current Opinions in Neurology,* 2010, 23: pp. 131–36; Herbert, "A Whole-Body Systems Approach to ASD," in *The Neuropsychology of Autism* (New York: Oxford University Press, 2011).

10   *What I found was that brains were larger:* Herbert, "Large brains in autism: The challenge of pervasive abnormality," *Neuroscientist,* 2005, 11: pp. 417–40; Herbert et al., "Dissociations of cerebral cortex, subcortical and cerebral white matter volumes in autistic boys," *Brain,* 2003, 126: pp. 1182–92; Herbert et al., "Localization of white matter volume increase in autism and developmental language disorder," *Annals of Neurology,* 2004, 55: pp. 499–510. See also Courchesne et al., "Brain growth across the lifespan in autism: age-specific changes in anatomical pathology," *Brain Research,* 2010, 1380: pp. 138–145.

10   *The psychologist Marcel Just:* Just et al., "Cortical activation and synchronization during sentence comprehension in high-functioning autism: Evidence of underconnectivity," *Brain,* 2004, 127: pp. 1811–21.

10   *Finally, in 2005, a research team:* Vargas et al., "Neuroglial activation and neuroinflammation in the brain of patients with autism," *Annals of Neurology,* 2005, 57: pp. 67–81.

10   *Other researchers were finding related immune problems:* Ashwood, Wills, and Van de Water, "The immune response in autism: A new frontier for autism research," *Journal of Leukocyte Biology,* 2006, 80: pp. 1–15.

11   *David Beversdorf, a pediatric neurologist:* Narayanan et al., "Effect of propranolol on functional connectivity in autism spectrum disorder—a pilot study," *Brain Imaging and Behavior,* 2010, 4: pp. 189–97.

12   *Some people want to blame rising autism:* Herbert, "Time to get a grip," *Autism Advocate,* 2006, 45: pp. 19–26, www.autism-society.org/site/Doc Server/eh_get_a_grip.pdf?docID=4821.

12   *these young bodies are pushed over an edge:* Herbert, "Autism: The centrality of active pathophysiology and the shift from static to chronic dynamic encephalopathy," in Chauhan, Chauhan, and Brown, *Autism: Oxidative Stress, Inflammation, and Immune Abnormalities* (Boca Raton, FL: Taylor & Francis/CRC Press, 2009), pp. 343–87.

20   *The financial costs alone of raising:* Ganz, "The lifetime distribution of the incremental societal costs of autism," *Archives of Pediatrics & Adolescent Medicine,* 2007, 161: pp. 343–49; Dawson, "The power of words: The IACC works to reconcile different perspectives on autism," *Autism Speaks Official Blog,* 2011, blog.autismspeaks.org/2011/01/20/iacc-the-power-of-words/.

21   *I believe that autism is not a genetic tragedy:* Herbert, "Learning from the autism catastrophe: Key leverage points," *Alternative Therapies in Health and Medicine,* 2008, 14: pp. 28–30.

CHAPTER 2. KNOW WHAT YOU CAN'T CONTROL—AND WHAT YOU CAN

26   *He then collected samples from 430 patients:* Talk given by Dr. Ivar Følling, son of Dr. Ivar Asbjørn Følling, presented at a meeting in Elsinore, Denmark, May 24–27, 1994, www.pkunews.org/about/history.

27   *And even in adults with PKU:* Snyderman, "Dietary and genetic therapy of inborn errors of metabolism: A summary," *Annals of the New York Academy of Sciences,* 1986, 477: pp. 231–36.

28   *Mark Bear, the MIT neuroscientist:* Interview with Karen Weintraub, Aug. 4, 2010, for article in *The Boston Globe.*

28   *The mice, which showed Rett symptoms:* Guy et al., "Reversal of neurological defects in a mouse model of Rett syndrome," *Science,* 2007, 315: pp. 1143–47.

29   *"Everyone assumes that autism, schizophrenia":* Carey Goldberg, "Autism-like disorder reversed in mice," *Boston Globe,* February 8, 2007.

29   *The first line of genetic testing:* Miller et al., "Consensus statement: Chromosomal microarray is a first-tier clinical diagnostic test for individuals

with developmental disabilities or congenital anomalies," *American Journal of Human Genetics,* 2010, 86: pp. 749–64.

30   **We now know that some children:** Sebat et al., "Strong association of de novo copy number mutations with autism," *Science,* 2007, 316: pp. 445–49; Eapen, "Genetic basis of autism: Is there a way forward?" *Current Opinions in Psychiatry,* 2011, 24: pp. 226–36.

30   **But one possibility is that these genetic mutations:** Kinney et al., "Environmental risk factors for autism: Do they help cause de novo genetic mutations that contribute to the disorder?" *Medical Hypotheses,* 2010, 74: pp. 102–6.

31   **Instead they have found hundreds of genes:** Betancur, "Etiological heterogeneity in autism spectrum disorders: More than 100 genetic and genomic disorders and still counting," *Brain Research,* 2011, 1380: pp. 42–77.

31   **Just for the record, there are more than five hundred:** Scriver, "The PAH gene, phenylketonuria, and a paradigm shift," *Human Mutation,* 2007, 28: pp. 831–45.

32   **Some genes, like the ones associated with fragile X:** Belmonte and Bourgeron, "Fragile X syndrome and autism at the intersection of genetic and neural networks," *Nature Neuroscience,* 2006, 9: pp. 1221–25.

32   **A recent autism twin study:** Hallmayer et al., Genetic Heritability and Shared Environmental Factors Among Twin Pairs with Autism. *Archives of General Psychiatry,* 2011, published online July 4, 2011.

32   **In a 1995 study of identical twins with schizophrenia:** Davis, Phelps, and Bracha, "Prenatal development of monozygotic twins and concordance for schizophrenia," *Schizophrenia Bulletin,* 1995, 21: pp. 357–66.

33   **When they gave up their native cooking:** Pratley, "Gene-environment interactions in the pathogenesis of type 2 diabetes mellitus: Lessons learned from the Pima Indians," *Proceedings of the Nutrition Society,* 1998, 57: pp. 175–81.

33   **Imagine a hill at the bottom of a lake:** After I wrote this metaphor I reviewed slides from past lectures by Sidney Baker, MD, some of which I'd heard, in which he uses a similar metaphor about hills under water. In his case the metaphor focuses on the increasing numbers in the population of more severe conditions like autism as compared to less severe conditions like attention deficit disorder, as environmental stress lowers the water level and exposes more vulnerabilities in the population. I am using the metaphor more to highlight how individual choices can make a difference in the water level for them and their children personally. I want to thank Dr. Baker for seeding this image in my mind.

34   **A fair number of rare metabolic disorders:** Zecavati and Spence, "Neurometabolic disorders and dysfunction in autism spectrum disorders," *Current Neurology and Neuroscience Reports,* 2009, 9: pp. 129–36.

35   *Researchers use the term* **allostatic load:** McEwen, "Stress, adaptation, and disease: Allostasis and allostatic load," *Annals of the New York Academy of Science,* 1998, 840: pp. 33–44; Glei et al., "Do chronic stressors lead to physiological dysregulation? Testing the theory of allostatic load," *Psychosomatic Medicine,* 2007, 69: pp. 769–76; Knox, "From 'omics' to complex disease: A systems biology approach to gene-environment interactions in cancer," *Cancer Cell International,* 2010, 10: pp. 1–13, www.cancerci.com/content/10/1/11.

37   *A new science of* "*nutrigenomics*"*:* Kaput, "Nutrigenomics research for personalized nutrition and medicine," *Current Opinions in Biotechnology,* 2008, 19: pp. 110–20.

37   *More and more scientists are calling for a move to:* Miller et al., "It is time for a positive approach to dietary guidance using nutrient density as a basic principle," *Journal of Nutrition,* 2009, 139: pp. 1198–1202; Krebs-Smith et al., "Americans do not meet federal dietary recommendations," *Journal of Nutrition,* 2010, 140: pp. 1832–38; Kant, "Consumption of energy-dense, nutrient-poor foods by adult Americans: Nutritional and health implications. The third National Health and Nutrition Examination Survey, 1988–1994," *American Journal of Clinical Nutrition,* 2000, 72: pp. 929–36.

38   *Let me quote Walter Willett:* Willett, *Eat, Drink, and Be Healthy: The Harvard Medical School Guide to Healthy Eating* (New York: Free Press, 2002), pp. 114–15.

39   *Zinc can enhance taste sensitivity:* Heckmann et al., "Zinc gluconate in the treatment of dysgeusia—a randomized clinical trial," *Journal of Dental Research,* 2005, 84: pp. 35–38.

41   *Even though there are upwards of eighty-five thousand chemicals:* Grandjean and Landrigan, "Developmental neurotoxicity of industrial chemicals," *Lancet,* 2006, 368: pp. 2167–78.

41   *Among the things you should know:* The Portal to Science, www.healthandenvironment.org/cgi-bin/portal.cgi, offers abundant references relevant to the points made on this list. See also Herbert, "Autism: The centrality of active pathophysiology and the shift from static to chronic dynamic encephalopathy," in Chauhan, Chauhan, and Brown, *Autism: Oxidative Stress, Inflammation, and Immune Abnormalities,* pp. 343–87.

42   *Toxins can also send confusing molecular signals:* T. Colburn, D. Dumanoski, and J. P. Meyers, *Our Stolen Future: Are We Threatening Our Fertility, Intelligence, and Survival? A Scientific Detective Story* (New York: Plume, 1997); S. Krimsky, *Hormonal Chaos: The Scientific and Social Origins of the Environmental Endocrine Hypothesis* (Baltimore: Johns Hopkins University Press, 1999).

43   *Children are generally exposed to more toxins:* Landrigan and Goldman, "Children's vulnerability to toxic chemicals: A challenge and opportunity to

strengthen health and environmental policy," *Health Affairs* (Millwood), 2011, 30: pp. 842–50.

43   *the precautionary principle:* The Wingspread Conference on the Precautionary Principle was convened by the Science and Environmental Health Network in 1998. Its conclusions can be found at www.sehn.org/precaution.html.

45   *Your child's vulnerability to bugs:* Dietert, "Distinguishing environmental causes of immune dysfunction from pediatric triggers of disease," *Open Pediatric Medicine Journal,* 2009, 3: pp. 38–44.

CHAPTER 3. REPAIR AND SUPPORT CELLS AND CYCLES

55   *Thousands of toxins, including chemicals and heavy metals:* Wallace and Starkov, "Mitochondrial targets of drug toxicity," *Annual Review of Pharmacology and Toxicology,* 2000, 40: pp. 353–88.

56   *While some of these problems may be caused by genes:* Giulivi et al., "Mitochondrial dysfunction in autism," *JAMA,* 2010, 304: pp. 2389–96. Zecavati and Spence also explored mitochondrial dysfunction in their paper "Neurometabolic disorders and dysfunction in autism spectrum disorders," *Current Neurology and Neuroscience Reports,* 2009, 9: pp. 129–36.

56   *Other studies have shown that mitochondria:* Wallace and Starkov, "Mitochondrial targets of drug toxicity," *Annual Review of Pharmacology and Toxicology,* 2000, 40: pp. 353–88.

56   *According to mitochondrial specialist John Jay Gargus:* Gargus, "Mitochondrial component of calcium signaling abnormality in autism," in Chauhan, Chauhan, and Brown, *Autism: Oxidative Stress, Inflammation, and Immune Abnormalities,* pp. 207–24.

56   *Researchers Daniel Rossignol and Richard Frye:* Rossignol and Frye, "Mitochondrial dysfunction in autism spectrum disorders: A systematic review and meta-analysis," *Molecular Psychiatry,* 2011, pp. 1–25.

58   *In 2008, researchers at the Massachusetts General:* Berk et al., "Glutathione: A novel treatment target in psychiatry," *Trends in Pharmacological Science,* 2008, 29: pp. 346–51.

58   *Oxidative stress is also present:* Stein et al., "Environmental threats to healthy aging, with a closer look at Alzheimer's and Parkinson's diseases," Greater Boston's Physicians for Social Responsibility and Science and Environmental Health Network, 2008, agehealthy.org/.

58   *Abha and Ved Chauhan and W. Ted Brown of the New York State Institute:* Chauhan, Chauhan, and Brown, *Autism: Oxidative Stress, Inflammation, and Immune Abnormalities;* Special Issue on Autism Spectrum Disorders, *American Journal of Biochemistry and Biotechnology* 4, no. 2: pp. 61–225, www.scipub.org/scipub/detail_issue.php?V_No=173&j_id=ajbb; Sajdel-Sulkowska et al., "Increase in cerebellar neurotrophin-3 and oxidative stress markers in autism," *Cerebellum,* Sept. 2009, vol. 8, pp. 366–72.

59   *Several studies have found markers of oxidative stress:* Ming et al., "Increased excretion of a lipid peroxidation biomarker in autism," *Prostaglandins Leukot Essent Fatty Acids,* 2005, 73: pp. 379–84; Yao et al., "Altered vascular phenotype in autism: Correlation with oxidative stress," *Archives of Neurology,* 2006, 63: pp. 1161–64.

59   *S. Jill James at the University of Arkansas:* James, "Oxidative stress and the metabolic pathology of autism," in Zimmerman, *Autism: Current Theories and Evidence* (Totowa, NJ: Humana Press, 2008), pp. 245–68.

60   *Research also shows that low methylation:* Zhang et al., "Dietary patterns are associated with levels of global genomic DNA methylation in a cancer-free population," *Journal of Nutrition,* 2011, pp. 1165–71.

64   *Here is a checklist (inspired by an article in the journal* Pediatrics*):* Kemper, Vohra, and Walls, American Academy of Pediatrics, "The use of complementary and alternative medicine in pediatrics," *Pediatrics,* 2008, 122: pp. 1374–86.

68   *There is some research suggesting NAC:* Lafleur et al., "N-acetylcysteine augmentation in serotonin reuptake inhibitor refractory obsessive-compulsive disorder," *Psychopharmacology* (Berlin), 2006, 184: pp. 254–56; Hardan et al., "A randomized controlled double-blind of N-acetylcysteine in children with autism," presentation, International Meeting for Autism Research, San Diego, May 2011.

70   *There are concerns that these technologies:* "PACE calls on governments to 'take all reasonable measures' to reduce exposure to electromagnetic fields," Parliamentary Assembly of the Council of Europe. Strasbourg, France, May 25, 2011. And Cai et al., "Frequency-modulated nuclear localization bursts coordinate gene regulation," *Nature,* 2008, 455: pp. 485–90.

72   *There is surprisingly little research:* Genuis, "Elimination of persistent toxicants from the human body," *Human & Experimental Toxicology,* 2011, 30: pp. 3–18.

73   *According to the U.S. Centers for Disease Control:* "Deaths associated with hypocalcemia from chelation therapy, Texas, Pennsylvania, and Oregon, 2003–2005," *Morbidity and Mortality Weekly Report,* March 3, 2006, 55, no. 8: pp. 204–7, www.cdc.gov/mmwr/preview/mmwrhtml/mm5508a3.htm.

73   *Standard medical practice is to use chelation for cases of extreme poisoning:* BlueCross BlueShield CareFirst Medical Policy: 2.01.027 Chelation Therapy, notesnet.carefirst.com/ecommerce/medicalpolicy.nsf/vwwebtablex/c53b4e 1e9fd79b67852577490043d151?OpenDocument.

CHAPTER 4. GET GUT AND IMMUNE SYSTEMS ON YOUR SIDE

78   *In late 2009, a panel of pediatric gastroenterologists:* Buie et al., "Evaluation, diagnosis, and treatment of gastrointestinal disorders in individuals with ASDs: A consensus report," *Pediatrics,* 2010, 125 Suppl 1: pp. S1–18; Buie et al., "Recommendations for evaluation and treatment of common

gastrointestinal problems in children with ASDs," *Pediatrics,* 2010, 125 Suppl 1: pp. S19–29.

78   ***The results, published in the journal*** Pediatrics: Campbell et al., "Distinct genetic risk based on association of MET in families with co-occurring autism and gastrointestinal conditions," *Pediatrics,* 2009, 123: pp. 1018–24.

79   ***Claudia Morris, a physician and researcher:*** Morris and Agin, "Syndrome of allergy, apraxia, and malabsorption: Characterization of a neurodevelopmental phenotype that responds to omega 3 and vitamin E supplementation," *Alternative Therapies in Health and Medicine,* 2009, 15: pp. 34–43.

81   ***According to extensive research by Alessio Fasano:*** Fasano, "Surprises from celiac disease," *Scientific American,* 2009, 301: pp. 54–61.

81   ***Although the gluten-free, casein-free (GFCF) diet:*** Whiteley et al., "The ScanBrit randomised, controlled, single-blind study of a gluten- and casein-free dietary intervention for children with autism spectrum disorders," *Nutritional Neuroscience,* 2010, 13: pp. 87–100.

82   ***Sulfur is needed to make the mucous lining:*** Alberti et al., "Sulphation deficit in 'low-functioning' autistic children: A pilot study," *Biological Psychiatry,* 1999, 46: pp. 420–24.

83   ***Jeff Gordon of Washington University in St. Louis:*** Reyes et al., "Viruses in the faecal microbiota of monozygotic twins and their mothers," *Nature,* 2010, 466: pp. 334–38; Turnbaugh et al., "A core gut microbiome in obese and lean twins," *Nature,* 2009, 457: pp. 480–84; Turnbaugh et al., "Organismal, genetic, and transcriptional variation in the deeply sequenced gut microbiomes of identical twins," *Proceedings of the National Academy of Sciences USA,* 2010, 107: pp. 7503–8; Turnbaugh et al., "The effect of diet on the human gut microbiome: A metagenomic analysis in humanized gnotobiotic mice," *Science Translational Medicine,* 2009, 1: p. 6ra14.

83   ***Gut bacteria can also affect your brain:*** Gonzalez et al., "The mind-body-microbial continuum," *Dialogues in Clinical Neuroscience,* 2011, 13: pp. 55–62; Collins and Bercik, "The relationship between intestinal microbiota and the central nervous system in normal gastrointestinal function and disease," *Gastroenterology,* 2009, 136: pp. 2003–14; Heijtz et al., "Normal gut microbiota modulates brain development and behavior," *Proceedings of the National Acadedmy of Sciences USA,* 2011, 108: pp. 3047–52.

83   ***In 2011, Antonio M. Persico and colleagues:*** Altieri et al., "Urinary p-cresol is elevated in small children with severe autism spectrum disorder," *Biomarkers* 2011, May, 16(3): pp. 252–60.

84   ***Jeremy Nicholson's research group at Imperial College:*** Yap et al., "Urinary metabolic phenotyping differentiates children with autism from their unaffected siblings and age-matched controls," *Journal of Proteome Research,* 2010, 9: pp. 2996–3004.

84   ***After finding abnormal clostridial bacteria:*** Finegold et al., "Gastrointestinal microflora studies in late-onset autism," *Clinical Infectious Diseases,*

2002, 35: pp. S6–16; Sandler et al., "Short-term benefit from oral vancomycin treatment of regressive-onset autism," *Journal of Child Neurology*, 2000, 15: pp. 429–35.

84   ***Researching mice, Derrick MacFabe:*** MacFabe et al., "Effects of the enteric bacterial metabolic product propionic acid on object-directed behavior, social behavior, cognition, and neuroinflammation in adolescent rats: Relevance to autism spectrum disorder," *Behavioural Brain Research*, 2011, 217: pp. 47–54.

86   ***What we do know is that everyone's immune:*** Dietert, "Developmental immunotoxicology (DIT): Windows of vulnerability, immune dysfunction and safety assessment," *Journal of Immunotoxicology*, 2008, 5: pp. 401–12; Hertz-Picciotto et al., "Prenatal exposures to persistent and non-persistent organic compounds and effects on immune system development," *Basic & Clinical Pharmacology & Toxicology*, 2008, 102: pp. 146–54.

86   ***Parents with an autoimmune disease:*** Atladottir et al., "Association of family history of autoimmune diseases and autism spectrum disorders," *Pediatrics*, 2009, 124: pp. 687–94.

86   ***Several researchers have shown that immune:*** Patterson, "Maternal infection and immune involvement in autism," *Trends in Molecular Medicine*, 2011, pp. 389–94; Shi et al., "Maternal influenza infection causes marked behavioral and pharmacological changes in the offspring," *Journal of Neuroscience*, 2003, 23: pp. 297–302.

86   ***Several studies have found that a number of mothers:*** Keil et al., "Parental autoimmune diseases associated with autism spectrum disorders in offspring," *Epidemiology*, 2010, 21: pp. 805–8; Atladottir et al., "Association of family history of autoimmune diseases and autism spectrum disorders," *Pediatrics*, 2009, 124: pp. 687–94; Mouridsen et al., "Autoimmune diseases in parents of children with infantile autism: A case-control study," *Developmental Medicine & Child Neurology*, 2007, 49: pp. 429–32.

86   ***In one 2010 study, a University of Puerto Rico:*** Dominguez-Bello et al., "Delivery mode shapes the acquisition and structure of the initial microbiota across multiple body habitats in newborns," *Proceedings of the National Academy of Sciences USA*, 2010, 107: pp. 11971–75.

86   ***During the earliest days of life, whatever bugs:*** Goodman et al., "Identifying genetic determinants needed to establish a human gut symbiont in its habitat," *Cell Host & Microbe*, 2009, 6: pp. 279–89; Eggesbo et al., "Development of gut microbiota in infants not exposed to medical interventions," *APMIS*, 2011, 119: pp. 17–35.

87   ***Preliminary research is suggesting that giving probiotics:*** Dotterud et al., "Probiotics in pregnant women to prevent allergic disease: A randomized, double-blind trial," *British Journal of Dermatology*, 2010, 163: pp. 616–23; Kopp and Salfeld, "Probiotics and prevention of allergic disease," *Current Opinion in Clinial Nutrition & Metabolic Care*, 2009, 12: pp. 298–303.

87   *Allergies can also deplete coenyzme Q10:* Miles et al., "Acquired coenzyme Q10 deficiency in children with recurrent food intolerance and allergies," *Mitochondrion,* 2011, 11: pp. 127–35.

88   *Autistic children also seem to have too many immune:* Ashwood et al., "Elevated plasma cytokines in autism spectrum disorders provide evidence of immune dysfunction and are associated with impaired behavioral outcome," *Brain, Behavior, and Immunity,* 2011, 25: pp. 40–45.

90   *It is now being studied as a possible treatment:* Zhou, Beevers, and Huang, "The targets of curcumin," *Current Drug Targets,* 2011, 12: pp. 332–47.

92   *According to one recent study, nearly 37 percent:* de Magistris et al., "Alterations of the intestinal barrier in patients with autism spectrum disorders and in their first-degree relatives," *Journal of Pediatric Gastroenterology and Nutrition,* 2010, 51: pp. 418–24.

92   *Thanks to the Autism Treatment Network:* Buie et al., "Evaluation, diagnosis, and treatment of gastrointestinal disorders in individuals with ASDs: a consensus report," *Pediatrics,* 2010, 125 Suppl 1: pp. S1–18; Buie et al., "Recommendations for evaluation and treatment of common gastrointestinal problems in children with ASDs," *Pediatrics,* 2010, 125 Suppl 1: pp. S19–29.

93   *A recent paper in* **The Lancet:** Pelsser et al., "Effects of a restricted elimination diet on the behaviour of children with attention-deficit hyperactivity disorder (INCA study): A randomised controlled trial," *Lancet,* 2011, 377: pp. 494–503.

94   *Sugar is junk food:* Taubes, "Is sugar toxic?" *New York Times Magazine,* April 13, 2011; Lustig, "The 'skinny' on childhood obesity: How our Western environment starves kids' brains," *Pediatric Annals,* 2006, 35: pp. 898–902, 905–7.

95   *A brief review of the problems with milk:* Oski, *Don't Drink Your Milk: The Frightening New Medical Facts about the World's Most Overrated Nutrient* (Brushton, NY: TEACH Services, 1996).

96   *Don't overlook the possibility that your child is sensitive:* Seroussi and Lewis, *The Encyclopedia of Dietary Interventions for the Treatment of Autism and Related Disorders* (Pennington, NJ: Sarpsborg Press, 2008).

98   *Once someone is sensitive and vulnerable:* Miller, "Toxicant-induced loss of tolerance," *Addiction,* 2001, 96: pp. 115–37.

98   *Pesticide residues are not good:* Roberts et al., "Maternal residence near agricultural pesticide applications and autism spectrum disorders among children in the California Central Valley," *Environmental Health Perspectives,* 2007, 115: pp. 1482–89; Rosas and Eskenazi, "Pesticides and child neurodevelopment," *Current Opinions in Pediatrics,* 2008, 20: pp. 191–97; Lu et al., "Dietary intake and its contribution to longitudinal organophosphorus pesticide exposure in urban/suburban children," *Environmental Health Perspectives,* 2008, 116: pp. 537–42.

100   *After years of assurances that food dyes:* Clinical Study from University

of Southampton School of Psychology Project Code T07040, Chronic and Acute Effects of Artificial Colourings and Preservatives on Children's Behaviour, Initial report from UK: www.food.gov.uk/multimedia/pdfs/additivesbehaviourfinrep.pdf; FDA valuation of this report: www.fda.gov/downloads/AdvisoryCommittees/CommitteesMeetingMaterials/FoodAdvisoryCommittee/UCM248110.pdf.

100 *One of food guru Michael Pollan's basic rules:* Pollan, *In Defense of Food* (New York: Penguin, 2009).

100 *In one experiment with mice, Ellen Silbergeld:* Via et al., "Low-dose exposure to inorganic mercury accelerates disease and mortality in acquired murine lupus," *Environmental Health Perspectives,* 2003, 111: pp. 1273–77.

101 *The Specific Carbohydrate Diet:* The diet is spelled out on several websites, including www.breakingtheviciouscycle.info/ and www.gapsdiet.com/.

101 *Naturally fermented foods, such as sauerkraut:* Gates and Schatz, *The Body Ecology Diet: Recovering Your Health and Rebuilding Your Immunity,* revised edition (Carlsbad, CA: Hay House, 2011); Fallon, *Nourishing Traditions* (Lanham, MD: New Trends, 1999); Katz, *Wild Fermentation: The Flavor, Nutrition, and Craft of Live-Culture Foods* (White River Junction, VT: Chelsea Green, 2003).

101 *All by themselves probiotics have not:* De Filippo et al., "Impact of diet in shaping gut microbiota revealed by a comparative study in children from Europe and rural Africa," *Proceedings of the National Academy of Sciences USA,* 2010, 107: pp. 14691–96; Romeo et al., "Immunomodulatory effect of fibres, probiotics and synbiotics in different life-stages," *Nutricion Hospitalaria,* 2010, 25: pp. 341–49.

103 *Researchers at the Mayo Clinic:* Poland and Oberg, "Vaccinomics and bioinformatics: Accelerants for the next golden age of vaccinology," *Vaccine,* 2010, 28: pp. 3509–10; Poland, "Vaccidents and adversomics," *Vaccine,* 2010, 28: pp. 6549–50; Haralambieva and Poland, "Vaccinomics, predictive vaccinology and the future of vaccine development," *Future Microbiology,* 2010, 5: pp. 1757–60; Poland, Ovsyannikova, and Jacobson, "Adversomics: The emerging field of vaccine adverse event immunogenetics," *Pediatric Infectious Disease Journal,* 2009, 28: pp. 431–32; "Application of pharmacogenomics to vaccines," *Pharmacogenomics,* 2009, 10: pp. 837–52; "Personalized vaccines: The emerging field of vaccinomics," *Expert Opinion on Biological Therapy,* 2008, 8: pp. 1659–67.

CHAPTER 5. HELP THE BODY MEND THE BRAIN

107 *She examined thirty children with autism and fever:* Curran et al., "Behaviors associated with fever in children with autism spectrum disorders," *Pediatrics,* 2007, 120: pp. e1386–92.

108 *In recent years, more and more neurologists:* Doidge, *The Brain That Changes Itself,* (New York: Penguin, 2007).

110 *Examining why children with autism have big brains:* Dager et al., "Imaging Evidence for Pathological Brain Development in Autism Spectrum Disorders." In Zimmerman, ed., *Autism: Current Theories and Evidence,* pp. 361–79.

111 *In epilepsy, when neurosurgeons remove a seizure "hot spot":* Hugg et al., "Normalization of contralateral metabolic function following temporal lobectomy demonstrated by 1H magnetic resonance spectroscopic imaging," *Annals of Neurology,* 1996, 40: pp. 236–69; Pan et al., "Neurometabolism in human epilepsy," *Epilepsia,* 2008, 49 Suppl 3: pp. 31–41; Serles et al., "Time course of postoperative recovery of N-acetyl-aspartate in temporal lobe epilepsy," *Epilepsia,* 2001, 42: pp. 190–97.

112 *As I mentioned in chapter 1, Dr. Carlos Pardo:* Vargas et al., "Neuroglial activation and neuroinflammation in the brain of patients with autism," *Annals of Neurology,* 2005, 57: pp. 67–81.

112 *Italian researchers Carla Lintas, Roberto Sacco:* Lintas, Sacco, and Persico, "Genome-wide expression studies in Autism spectrum disorder, Rett syndrome, and Down syndrome," *Neurobiology of Disease,* in press.

113 *But as R. Douglas Fields explains in:* Fields, *The Other Brain: From Dementia to Schizophrenia, How New Discoveries About the Brain are Revolutionizing Medicine and Science* (New York: Simon & Schuster, 2009). Also Barres, "The Mystery and Magic of Glia: a perspective on their roles in health and disease." *Neuron,* 2008, 60: pp. 430–40.

113 *In the genetic disease Huntington's:* Hsiao and Chern, "Targeting glial cells to elucidate the pathogenesis of Huntington's disease," *Molecular Neurobiology,* 2010, 41: pp. 248–55.

115 *Third, astrocytes maintain brain health:* Aschner et al., "Glial cells in neurotoxicity development," *Annual Review of Pharmacology and Toxicology,* 1999, 39: pp. 151–73; Aschner et al., "Methylmercury alters glutamate transport in astrocytes," *Neurochemistry International,* 2000, 37: pp. 199–206.

116 *Liver cells are the trash collectors:* Phone interview with Michael Aschner, Feb. 8, 2011.

116 *Michael Gershon of Columbia University:* Gershon, *The Second Brain: A Groundbreaking New Understanding of Nervous Disorders of the Stomach and Intestine* (New York: Harper, 1999).

116 *Though we barely knew about them a decade ago:* Savidge, Sofroniew, and Neunlist, "Starring roles for astroglia in barrier pathologies of gut and brain," *Laboratory Investigation,* 2007, 87: pp. 731–36; Ruhl, "Glial cells in the gut," *Neurogastroenterology & Motility,* 2005, 17: pp. 777–90.

118 *"It's going to continue unimpeded":* Phone interview with Michael Aschner, Feb. 8, 2011.

118 *In a review published in 2008, Christopher Moore:* Lecrux and Hamel, "The neurovascular unit in brain function and disease," *Acta Physiologica* (Ox-

ford), 2011, pp. 47–69; Moore and Cao, "The hemo-neural hypothesis: On the role of blood flow in information processing," *Journal of Neurophysiology*, 2008, 99: pp. 2035–47; Herbert, "Autism: The centrality of active pathophysiology and the shift from static to chronic dynamic encephalopathy," in Chauhan, Chauhan, and Brown, *Autism: Oxidative Stress, Inflammation, and Immune Abnormalities*, pp. 343–87.

122 ***Researchers at the University of Oklahoma:*** Hunter et al., "Neuroligin-deficient mutants of *C. elegans* have sensory processing deficits and are hypersensitive to oxidative stress and mercury toxicity," *Disease Models & Mechanisms*, 2010, 3: pp. 366–76.

124 ***Studies show that fish oil supplementation:*** Huss, Volp, and Stauss-Grabo, "Supplementation of polyunsaturated fatty acids, magnesium and zinc in children seeking medical advice for attention-deficit/hyperactivity problems—an observational cohort study," *Lipids in Health and Disease*, 2010, 9: p. 105.

124 ***Research is mixed, though a fair number of studies:*** Mousain-Bosc et al., "Improvement of neurobehavioral disorders in children supplemented with magnesium-vitamin B6. II. Pervasive developmental disorder-autism," *Magnesium Research*, 2006, 19: pp. 53–62.

124 ***More GABA means better brakes:*** Office of Dietary Supplements, National Institutes of Health: ods.od.nih.gov/factsheets/VitaminB6-HealthProfessional/#h2.

125 ***Terbutaline, used to treat lung diseases:*** Kilburn, Thrasher, and Immers, "Do terbutaline- and mold-associated impairments of the brain and lung relate to autism?" *Toxicology and Industrial Health*, 2009, 25: pp. 703–10; Aldridge et al., "Developmental exposure to terbutaline and chlorpyrifos: Pharmacotherapy of preterm labor and an environmental neurotoxicant converge on serotonergic systems in neonatal rat brain regions," *Toxicology and Applied Pharmacology*, 2005, 203: pp. 132–44.

125 ***Toxins like mercury can clearly accumulate:*** Aschner et al., "Methylmercury alters glutamate transport in astrocytes," *Neurochemistry International*, 2000, 37: pp. 199–206.

127 ***Even if the infection is milder, like the flu:*** Patterson, "Maternal infection and immune involvement in autism," *Trends in Molecular Medicine*, 2011, pp. 389–94; Fatemi, "Multiple pathways in prevention of immune-mediated brain disorders: Implications for the prevention of autism," *Journal of Neuroimmunology*, 2009, 217: pp. 8–9; Fatemi et al., "Maternal infection leads to abnormal gene regulation and brain atrophy in mouse offspring: Implications for genesis of neurodevelopmental disorders," *Schizophrenia Research*, 2008, 99: pp. 56–70.

127 ***Some bugs soak up and hang on to toxins:*** Boyd, "Heavy metal pollutants and chemical ecology: Exploring new frontiers," *Journal of Chemical Ecology*, 2010, 36: pp. 46–58.

CHAPTER 6. CALM BRAIN CHAOS

134   *No one knows for sure what the low sensitivity is about:* Tordjman et al., "Pain reactivity and plasma beta-endorphin in children and adolescents with autistic disorder," PloS One, 2009, 4: p. e5289.

136   *You can also help your child:* Myles, Adreon, and Gitlitz, *Simple Strategies That Work! Helpful Hints for All Educators of Students* (Overland Park, KS: Autism Asperger Publishing, 2006), p. 30.

136   *In 2003 researchers John Rubenstein and Michael Merzenich:* Rubenstein and Merzenich, "Model of autism: Increased ratio of excitation/inhibition in key neural systems," *Genes, Brain and Behavior,* 2003, 2: pp. 255–67.

136   *In late 2010 researchers:* Markram and Markram, "The intense world theory—a unifying theory of the neurobiology of autism," *Frontiers in Human Neuroscience,* 2010, 4: p. 224.

137   *Mark Bear's theory of fragile X has similarities:* Bear, Huber, and Warren, "The mGluR theory of fragile X mental retardation," *Trends in Neuroscience,* 2004, 27: pp. 370–77.

137   *The cerebellum is also the part of the brain:* Courchesne et al., "Unusual brain growth patterns in early life in patients with autistic disorder: An MRI study," *Neurology,* 2001, 57: pp. 245–54.

138   *The writer Tito Rajarshi Mukhopadhyay:* Mukhopadhyay, *How Can I Talk If My Lips Don't Move? Inside My Autistic Mind* (New York: Arcade, 2008), p. 1.

139   *One recent study estimated that 60–70 percent:* Goldman et al., "Motor stereotypes in children with autism and other developmental disorders," *Developmental Medicine & Child Neurology,* 2009, 51: pp. 30–38.

140   *About 80 percent of children and adolescents with autism:* Oyane and Bjorvatn, "Sleep disturbances in adolescents and young adults with autism and Asperger syndrome," *Autism,* 2005, 9: pp. 83–94; Liu et al., "Sleep disturbances and correlates of children with autism spectrum disorders," *Child Psychiatry and Human Development,* 2006, 37: pp. 179–91.

141   *Getting* regular exercise *every day:* www.mypyramid.gov/pyramid/physical _activity_amount.html.

142   *There is a fair amount of research on melatonin:* Melke et al., "Abnormal melatonin synthesis in autism spectrum disorders," *Molecular Psychiatry,* 2008, 13: pp. 90–98; Chaste et al., "Identification of pathway-biased and deleterious melatonin receptor mutants in autism spectrum disorders and in the general population," PLoS One, 2010, 5: p. e11495.

142   *Night terrors, though terrifying for you:* Here's one reference about night terrors from the Mayo Clinic: ip-24-248-24-17.coxfiber.net/health_reference/ Childrens-Health/DS01016.cfm.

143   *Studies find seizure activity:* Spence and Schneider, "The role of epilepsy and epileptiform EEGs in autism spectrum disorders," *Pediatric Research,* 2009, 65: pp. 599–606.

143 *A much larger proportion of children:* Ibid.

144 *Frances Jensen, of Children's Hospital Boston:* Jensen, "Epilepsy as a spectrum disorder: Implications from novel clinical and basic neuroscience," *Epilepsia,* 2011, 52 Suppl 1: pp. 1–6.

144 *Scientists are starting to find overlap:* Tuchman, Moshe, and Rapin, "Convulsing toward the pathophysiology of autism," *Brain Development,* 2009, 31: pp. 95–103.

144 *The more excitable brain cells are:* Riazi, Galic, and Pittman, "Contributions of peripheral inflammation to seizure susceptibility: Cytokines and brain excitability," *Epilepsy Research,* 2010, 89: pp. 34–42.

146 *There is some evidence that various nondrug approaches:* Gaby, "Natural approaches to epilepsy," *Alternative Medicine Review,* 2007, 12: pp. 9–24; Frye et al., "Traditional and non-traditional treatments for autism spectrum disorder with seizures: An on-line survey," *BMC Pediatrics* 2011, vol. 11, pp. 37–55, www.biomedcentral.com/1471-2431/11/37.

147 *There is a small amount of literature:* Frymann, Carney, and Springall, "Effect of osteopathic medical management on neurologic development in children," *Journal of the American Osteopathic Association,* 1992, 92: pp. 729–44; Frymann, *The Osteopathic Approach to Children with Seizure Disorders: Complementary and Alternative Therapies for Epilepsy* (New York: Demos Medical Publishing, 2005), pp. 273–84.

149 *One teenager with autism, named Carly Fleischmann:* John McKinsey, "Breakthrough: Autistic Teen Finds Voice," ABC News, Feb. 20, 2009.

150 *Michael Merzenich, a professor of neuroscience:* Wolman, "The Truth About Autism: Scientists Reconsider What They Think They Know," *Wired,* Feb. 25, 2008.

150 *That's basically what a group of Canadian researchers:* Dawson et al., "The level and nature of autistic intelligence," *Psychological Science,* 2007, 18: pp. 657–62.

153 *In one example I heard about recently:* Kluth, *You're Going to Love This Kid* (Baltimore: Paul H. Brookes, 2003), p. 111.

153 *Scientists from MIT have been developing technologies:* Rosenbaum, "High-Tech Clues to Facial Cues," *Boston Globe,* Oct. 27, 2008.

154 *Judy Endow writes about:* Endow, *Practical Solutions for Stabilizing Students with Classic Autism to Be Ready to Learn in Rhode Island: Getting to Go!* (Overland Park, KS: Autism Asperger Publishing, 2010), p. 35.

154 *The Groden Center in Rhode Island:* Conversation with June Groden, March 14, 2011.

CHAPTER 7. JOIN YOUR CHILD'S WORLD

165 *A psychologist, Carr helped develop:* Carr et al., "Positive behavior support: Evolution of an applied science," *Journal of Positive Behavioral Interventions,* 2002, 4: pp. 4–16; Carr and Durand, "Reducing behavior problems through

functional communication training," *Journal of Applied Behavioral Analysis,* 1985, 18: pp. 111–26.

166 ***In her wonderful memoir,* Strange Son:** Iversen, *Strange Son* (New York: Riverhead, 2006), pp. 302–4.

167 ***Dr. Carr and I wrote a paper together:*** Carr and Herbert, "Integrating behavioral and biomedical approaches: A marriage made in heaven," *Autism Advocate,* April 2008, pp. 46–52.

170 ***The Ziggurat Model is an approach:*** Aspy and Grossman, *The Ziggurat Model: A Framework for Designing Comprehensive Interventions for Individuals with High-Functioning Autism and Asperger Syndrome* (Overland Park, KS: Autism Asperger Publishing, 2007).

170 ***The Comprehensive Autism Planning System (CAPS):*** Henry and Myles, *The Comprehensive Autism Planning System (CAPS) for Individuals with Asperger Syndrome, Autism and Related Disabilities: Integrating Best Practices Throughout the Student's Day* (Overland Park, KS: Autism Asperger Publishing, 2007).

172 ***She describes the meltdown process as a train with four cars:*** Judy Endow, *Outsmarting Explosive Behavior: A Visual System of Support and Intervention for Individuals with Autism Spectrum Disorders* (Overland Park, KS: Autism Asperger Publishing, 2009).

174 ***According to educator Brenda Smith Myles, there is a "hidden curriculum":*** Myles, Trautman, and Schelvan, *The Hidden Curriculum: Practical Solutions for Understanding Unstated Rules in Social Situations* (Overland Park, KS: Autism Asperger Publishing, 2004); Endow, *Hidden Curriculum One-a-Day Calendar for Older Adolescents and Adults* (Overland Park, KS: Autism Asperger Publishing, 2010 and 2011).

178 ***The Incredible 5-Point Scale, developed by Kari Dunn Buron:*** www.5point scale.com/.

179 ***Researchers Rosalind Picard and Matthew Goodwin:*** Goodwin, Velicer, and Intille, "Telemetric monitoring in the behavior sciences," *Behavior Research Methods,* 2008, 40: pp. 328–41.

179 ***June Groden, cofounder of the Groden Center:*** www.grodencenter.org/ publications-and-research/publications.

180 ***Groden's latest book and work at the center:*** Groden, Kantor, and Cooper, *How Everyone on the Autism Spectrum, Young and Old, Can: Become Resilient, Be More Optimistic, Enjoy Humor, Be Kind, and Increase Self-efficacy: A Positive Psychology Approach* (London: Jessica Kingsley, 2011).

180 ***Though we can't know for sure what helped:*** www.autismtreatmentcenter .org/.

CHAPTER 8. FROM AUTISTIC TO EXTRAORDINARY

187 ***Melody says she was completely perplexed:*** Greene, *The Explosive Child: A New Approach for Understanding and Parenting Easily Frustrated, Chronically Inflexible Children* (New York: Harper 2010).

CHAPTER 9. LEAD THE REVOLUTION!

210   *Charles Scriver, a world-renowned pediatrician and geneticist:* Scriver, "The PAH gene, phenylketonuria, and a paradigm shift," *Human Mutation,* 2007, 28: pp. 831–45.

215   *The National Institute of Mental Health is conducting:* "Identification of Characteristics Associated with Symptom Remission in Autism, Protocol Number: 09-M-0171," clinicalstudies.info.nih.gov/cgi/wais/bold032001.pl ?A_09-M-0171.html@Autism.

217   *The Autism Research Institute has created a treatment checklist:* www .autism.com/ind_atec_survey.asp.

217   *It now has some published scientific support:* Magiati et al., "Is the Autism Treatment Evaluation Checklist a useful tool for monitoring progress in children with autism spectrum disorders?" *Journal of Intellectual Disability Research,* 2011, 55: pp. 302–12.

CHAPTER 10. DO IT FOR YOURSELF, YOUR NEXT BABY, YOUR FAMILY, AND YOUR WORLD

225   *One study showed that parents diagnosed with schizophrenia:* Daniels et al., "Parental psychiatric disorders associated with autism spectrum disorders in the offspring," *Pediatrics,* 2008, 121: pp. e1357–62.

227   *For women not taking prenatal vitamins:* Schmidt et al., "Prenatal vitamins, one-carbon metabolism gene variants, and risk for autism," *Epidemiology,* 2011, 22: pp. 476–85.

228   *One recent study showed that women who took 4,000 IU a day:* Wagner et al., "Vitamin D Supplementation during Pregnancy Part 2 NICHD/CTSA Randomized Clinical Trial (RCT): Outcomes," paper presented at the Pediatric Academic Societies annual meeting in Vancouver, British Columbia, Canada, May 2010.

230   *There's some new research suggesting that the timing of when:* Tanpowpong et al., "Season of Birth and Celiac Disease in Massachusetts Children," paper presented May 8, 2011, at Digestive Disease Week, Chicago, suggesting that babies born in spring and summer were more likely to have celiac. Authors hypothesize that this may be because spring/summer babies are introduced to gluten in the winter, when cold season is at its height, and the combination may lead to celiac.

231   *Probiotics may also be helpful for maintaining:* Dupont et al., "Alpha-lactalbumin-enriched and probiotic-supplemented infant formula in infants with colic: Growth and gastrointestinal tolerance," *European Journal of Clinical Nutrition,* 2010, 64: pp. 765–67; Kukkonen et al., "Long-term safety and impact on infection rates of postnatal probiotic and prebiotic (synbiotic) treatment: Randomized, double-blind, placebo-controlled trial," *Pediatrics,* 2008, 122: pp. 8–12; Savino and Tarasco, "New treatments for infant

colic," *Current Opinion in Pediatrics,* 2010, pp. 791–97; Thomas and Greer, "Probiotics and prebiotics in pediatrics," *Pediatrics,* 2010, 126: pp. 1217–31.

231   *However, at this point pediatricians are not advised:* Johnson and Myers, "Identification and evaluation of children with autism spectrum disorders," *Pediatrics,* 2007, 120: pp. 1183–215.

236   *Mother (and father, too) can get "in synch":* Reyna and Pickler, "Mother-infant synchrony," *Journal of Obstetric Gynecologic Neonatal Nursing,* 2009, 38: pp. 470–77; Feldman, "Parent-infant synchrony and the construction of shared timing: Physiological precursors, developmental outcomes, and risk conditions," *Journal of Child Psychology and Psychiatry,* 2007, 48: pp. 329–54.

240   *A study in the journal* **Pediatrics:** Dawson et al., "Randomized, controlled trial of an intervention for toddlers with autism: The Early Start Denver Model," *Pediatrics,* 2010, 125: pp. e17–23.

242   *The United Nations released a report in 2011:* United Nations Special Rapporteur on the Right to Food, Agro-cology and the Right to Food, 2011, www.srfood.org/index.php/en/component/content/article/1-latest-news/1174-report-agroecology-and-the-right-to-food.

242   *Some people even describe the plant foods:* Junger, *Clean: The Revolutionary Program to Restore the Body's Natural Ability to Heal Itself* (New York: Harper One, 2010) p. 87.

INDEX

Note: * = Name changed to protect privacy.

digestive system (*cont'd*)
esophagus, 80
and food, 90–98, 211–12
gastrointestinal distress, 77–79, 82–84
gut-blood barrier, 109
gut bugs, 82–84, 100–102
and immune system, 85
large intestine, 82
leaky gut, 92, 117
mouth, 79–80
self-restricted diets, 92–97
small intestine, 80–82
stomach, 80
and stress, 104–5
tests of, 91–92
and toxins, 98–100
directions, following, 14
Discrete Trial teaching, 174, 175
dishwashers, 239
DNA, 29
and amino acids, 55
and folinic acid, 69
and mutation, 30
doctors:
locating, 195
tips for, 261–63
whole-body training of, 217
Down syndrome, 112, 201
drawing, 200–201
drugs, side effects of, 55, 82
dynamic encephalopathy, 108
dysbiosis, 83
dysfunction, gray zone of, 110–11, 118,
125, 144, 147
dyspraxia, 63, 79

ears, inflammation of, 88
EarthEasy.com, 44
echolalia, 135, 152–53
EEG (electroencephalogram), 143–44,
145, 146, 150–51
Egeland, Borgny, 26
Egeland, Dag, 26
eggs, as potential allergen, 231
elective surgery, 229
electrodermal activity, 179
electromagnetic frequencies, 70–71
electronic diaries, 214
electron transport chain, 55

emotions, 169, 173
encephalopathy, 108
endocrine disrupters, 42–43
Endow, Judy, 135, 154, 161–62, 164, 198,
207
on focusing, 174
on meltdowns, 172–73
*Practical Solutions for Stabilizing
Students,* 172
on sensory breaks, 171, 173
and yoga, 181
energy supply, 121
environment, 14, 208
and behavior, 166, 169
and chronic illness, 64
external, 166–67
and free radicals, 57–58
and gene expression, 31
and genetic mutations, 30
and genetic variations, 33, 122–23
interests, 167
internal, 167–69
and mitochondrial problems, 56–57
patterns in, 173–74
and risk factors, 33, 46–47
sensory overload, 166
social triggers, 166
stabilization, 171–73
toxins in, 59
uterine, 32
your control over, 34–35
Environmental Working Group, 44
enzymes, 55, 80, 97–98
epigenetic modifications, 31
epilepsy, 111, 131, 143–47, 151
epilepsy spectrum disorder, 144
Epsom salt baths, 65, 134, 142
Equal, 99, 141
esophagus, 80
essential fatty acids, 69, 104, 124, 149,
227, 231
eustachian tubes, 88
excitation, 115, 136, 138, 143, 144
excitotoxins, 99, 118, 123
exercise:
and self-control, 171–72
and sleep, 141
soreness from, 54
and stress, 172

expectations:
  and anxiety, 194
  vs. reality, 154
eye contact, 235–36

facial expressions, 153
FAD molecules, 55
Fasano, Alessio, 81
fatigue, 169
feelings, 14, 131, 202
feet, cold water on, 142
Feldenkrais, Moshe, 197
Feldenkrais Method, 139, 196–97
fermented foods, 101
fertilizers, chemical, 97, 242
fever:
  children emerging from autism during, 106–7, 119
  effects on brain, 107
fiber, 36, 82, 101
Fields, R. Douglas, *The Other Brain,* 113
fight-or-flight response, 104, 128
Finegold, Sydney, 84
fish, mercury in, 100, 125
fish oil, 98, 124, 146, 226, 231
Five-Point Scale, 178
flame retardants, 42
flavonoids, 37
Fleischmann, Carly, 149–50
Floortime, 177
FMRP, 28
focus:
  intense, 131, 154–55
  on salient information, 174
folate, 57, 229
folic acid, 146, 227
folinic acid, 69
Følling, Ivar Asbjørn, 26–27
food, 35–41
  allergies to, 78, 79, 80, 91, 142, 168–69
  and the brain, 123–25, 212
  and cells, 211
  chewing, 79, 80
  child-friendly recipes, 39
  cultured, 101
  daily log of, 39, 90, 100, 251–52
  and digestive system, 90–98, 211–12
  fermented, 101
  and genes, 36–37, 212

high-quality, 90
how to get started, 38–40
and immune system, 90–98
introduction of, 175–76
inventory of, 38–39
junk food, 37–38, 39, 84, 94, 95, 124, 241
labels on packages of, 37
and mitochondria, 55
organic, 98–99
picky eaters, 79, 97, 175–76
plant-based, 37–38
and pregnancy, 227–28
processed, 38, 124
purees, 39, 40–41
reactions to, 213
Recommended Daily Allowance (RDA), 36, 68
sensitivities, 96–97, 168–69
shelf life of, 38
too much, 53–54
toxins in, 45, 228–29
see also diet
food anxiety, 175
food challenge test for allergies, 91
food dyes, 100, 124, 141
fragile X syndrome, 6, 28, 32, 137, 225
Franklin, Cindy*, 130, 147, 148, 152
Franklin, Jimmy*:
  and autism triggers, 131–32, 149, 165, 166
  clumsiness of, 137
  and dietary changes, 142, 152
  hope for future, 207
  insensitivity to pain and cold, 134–35
  not talking, 148–49, 152
  repetitive movements of, 139
  and seizures, 130, 147
free radicals, 57–58
friendship, 200
fruits and vegetables:
  antioxidants in, 58
  cruciferous, 70
  fiber in, 101
  high nutrient density in, 37–38
  magnesium in, 134
  phytonutrients in, 37, 39

and precautionary principle, 43–44
and pregnancy, 125, 127, 228–29
and stress, 45–46
toxoplasmosis, 127, 230
transcendence, blockage to, 15
TRANSCEND research program, 145
transition reaction, 213
trauma, and blood-brain barrier, 109
treatment log, 253–54
treatment options:
checklist of, 64–65, 217
control of, 208–9
treatment successes, 211–13, 215
triggers:
of autism, 131–32
of cancer, 88
of seizures, 131, 165, 166
tropical diseases, 229
turmeric, 89
twin studies, 32
Tylenol, 104
tyrosine, 27

ulcerative colitis, 101, 102
ultrasound, 229
underconnectivity, 10, 115
uterine environment, 32

vaccinations, 102–4, 237–38
vaccines, preservative-free, 104
vaccinomics, 103
vaginal delivery, 86
valproate, 136
vancomycin, 84
vegetables, *see* fruits and vegetables
vegetarian diet, 82
verbal apraxia, 149–50
vestibular sense, 171
villi, 80–81
viruses, 45
and mitochondria, 55–56
vision:
building, 21
description of, 23–24
visual information, 173
visual problems, 152
vitamin A, 69, 98
vitamin B complex, 55, 57, 66, 69, 82, 124–25, 146, 226, 228

vitamin C, 57–58
vitamin D, 69, 98, 146, 227–28
vitamin E, 57, 69, 79, 149
vitamins, 36–37
and the brain, 123
and enzymes, 55
in fruits and vegetables, 39
for infants, 231
methylated, 228
multivitamins, 39–40, 66–69
prenatal, 227
Vitamix, 39, 40, 239
vulnerability, 12
to bugs, 45
environmental, 122–23
metabolic, 36
in pregnancy, 225–30
to toxic exposure, 43
water filters, 44
water quality, 44
weak central coherence, 133, 136
web:
body, 16
brain, 16
list of characteristics and symptoms, 21–23
strengthening, 18–19
what you can do, 21–25
see also whole-body method
Wechsler Intelligence Scale, 150
white matter, 10
whole-body method, 19–20, 156, 224
brain measures, 214
community-based research, 215
comparative effectiveness research, 215
doctor training in, 217
grassroots science, 216–17
multivariate longitudinal design, 214
and PKU, 27–28
regluing the brain, 123
and regression, 119–20
reverse-engineered, 215
and seizures, 146
statistical methods, 214–15
studying problems via, 7, 9, 10, 11, 16–17, 52, 118–20
summary, 255–60
and systems biology, 213–14
systems science, 213–15

ABOUT THE AUTHORS

MARTHA HERBERT, MD, PHD, is an assistant professor of neurology at Harvard Medical School and a pediatric neurologist at Massachusetts General Hospital, where she is the director of the TRANSCEND research program. She sits on the Scientific Advisory Committee for Autism Speaks.

KAREN WEINTRAUB, MA, is an award-winning journalist and freelance health writer for outlets like *The Boston Globe, USA Today,* and the BBC. A past recipient of a prestigious Knight Center for Science Journalism fellowship, she also teaches journalism at the Harvard Extension School and Boston University.

ABOUT THE TYPE

This book was set in Minion, a 1990 Adobe Originals typeface by Robert Slimbach. Minion is inspired by classical, old-style typefaces of the late Renaissance, a period of elegant, beautiful, and highly readable type designs. Created primarily for text setting, Minion combines the aesthetic and functional qualities that make text type highly readable with the versatility of digital technology.